First Aid: Contemporary Practices and Principles

First Aid: Contemporary Practices and Principles

Edited by **Brent Q. Hafen**
Alton L. Thygerson
Ray A. Petersen
Brigham Young University
Provo, Utah

BURGESS PUBLISHING COMPANY • Minneapolis, Minnesota 55415

Copyright © 1972 by Burgess Publishing Company
Printed in the United States of America
SBN 8087-0837-6
Library of Congress Catalog Card Number 72-82623

2   3   4   5   6   7   8   9

Preface

This volume is a collection of articles on first aid. The selected readings represent a search of all available literature on first aid. The articles present recently established procedures and significant concepts that are of importance to today's first aider but are often difficult to locate and obtain. As the literature was reviewed it became increasingly clear that articles are very scant in some areas of first aid; therefore, some original writing by the editors was necessary to support these areas. All selections were made on the basis of practical applicability and significance of ideas.

The purpose of this book is to provide concepts and principles which are not often found in existing first aid textbooks. This book is designed to supplement and complement rather than duplicate present texts on first aid such as the *American Red Cross First Aid Textbook.* Thus, articles dealing with common concepts, i.e., shock, wounds, fractures, bandaging, etc., were intentionally excluded.

Our thanks go to the authors and publishers who have permitted us to reprint their work.

Brent Q. Hafen
Alton L. Thygerson
Ray A. Petersen

Contents

Section I

Introduction

Trauma—A National Problem

Penalty of Progress

Man has a persistent tendency to tamper with his environment and to live in an environment of his own making without sufficient attention to the consequences. The complexity of the public health problems today is due to man's alteration of his environment and to a larger proportion of man-made health issues. The greatest threat lies in the expansion of our intellectual activity itself. We are pressured by our own biologic success. Though newspapers may highlight deaths due to tornadoes in the Middle West or hurricanes in the South, the grim fact is that on any weekend more persons are killed on the highways by motor vehicles than are killed by the total forces of nature.

A major obstacle to progress has often been the tendency to regard a given problem, whatever its nature, as unconquerable (1). This has also been the case with accidents. Public opinion, not only in the United States but throughout the civilized world, has tended to regard accidents as unfortunate occurrences to be accepted as inevitable. Those responsible for safeguarding the public health cannot accept the more than 116,000 deaths and 10,000,000 disabling injuries which are now occurring every year without intensifying their efforts to reduce this constant tragic loss to society. In the United States today, during the period from the first year of life to the age of thirty-five, more deaths result from accidental injury than from any other cause.

In order to better appreciate the magnitude of this national problem, the following summary is reproduced directly (Figure 1).

Cost to the Nation

The toll in 1970 from all accidents was 113,000 persons killed and 10,800,000 injured; per 100,000 persons, the death rate was 57.4 percent which was down 2 percent from 1969. Of the principal classes of accidents contributing to these deaths, 49 percent of these deaths were associated with a motor vehicle, 12 percent with work, 23 percent with the home, and 16 percent with recreation, transportation besides motor vehicles, public building accidents, and the like. Male deaths outnumbered female deaths by approximately 2 to 1.

In 1968, disabling injuries were reported at 11,000,000 by the National Safety Council, and previous experience would indicate that approximately

Reprinted from *Status of Research in Trauma and the Critically Injured*, a report by the Surgery Training Committee of the National Institute of General Medical Sciences, 1970, Public Health Service, U.S. Department of Health, Education and Welfare.

The National Accident Fatality Toll

	1970	1969	Change
ALL ACCIDENTS	113,000	115,000	— 2 %
Motor-vehicle	55,300	56,400	— 2 %
Public non-motor-vehicle	20,000	21,000	— 5 %
Home	27,000	27,000	0 %
Work	14,200	14,200	0 %

Note: The motor-vehicle totals include some deaths also included in work and home. This duplication amounted to about 3,500 in 1970 and 3,600 in 1969. All figures are National Safety Council estimates.

All Accidents

Killed—113,000, down 2 per cent from 1969.

Injured—10,800,000.

Cost—$26,000,000,000. Includes wage loss, medical expense, administrative and claim settlement costs of insurance for all accidents, certain "indirect" costs of work accidents, and property damage in traffic accidents and fires.

Deaths of children under 5 years decreased about 4 per cent in 1970. Among children 5-14 years old the death total was down 1 per cent. Adult group changes were: 15-24 years, down 2 per cent; 25-44 and 45-64 years, unchanged; 65-74 years, up 1 per cent, and 75 years and older, down 6 per cent.

Fatal falls 18,300, down 4 per cent from 1969; drownings 7,200, down 1 per cent. Fires, burns and drownings showed no change. Poisoning by solids and liquids, up 12 per cent from 1969.

The 1970 death rate per 100,000 population was 55.5, down 3 per cent from 57.0 in 1969.

Work Accidents

Killed—14,200. This was unchanged from the 1969 total.

Injured—2,200,000.

Cost—$9,000,000,000. Includes certain "indirect" costs of work accidents, as well as wage loss, medical expense and the administrative and claim settlement costs of insurance, and loss from business fires. Not included is the value of property damage in noninjury accidents other than fires and the indirect losses of all fires.

Total all-industry employment was up less than 1 per cent from 1969.

Worker Accidents

Killed—56,400, down 400 from 1969. On job, 14,200; off job, 42,200.

Injured—5,300,000.

Time lost, including indirect, amounted to more than 250 million man-days, equivalent to the shut-down of plants with more than 1 million workers for one year.

Public Accidents

(Not Motor Vehicle)

Killed—20,000, down 1,000 from 1969.

Injured—2,600,000.

Cost—$1,400,000,000.

Deaths decreased in the 5-14-year age group. There were increases for children under 5 years of age and for the 15-24-year age group; decreases occurred in all other age groups. There was an increase in water transport deaths and decreases in air transport, fires, burns, drowning, firearms and falls.

Railroad Accidents

Yearly totals are not available, but in the first five months of 1970, the Federal Railroad Administration reported 540 highway grade crossing fatalities, compared with 607 during the same months of 1969. Reports from state motor vehicle departments indicate a full year total of about 1,480 deaths compared with about 1,500 in the previous year.

Airplane Accidents

There were no deaths of passengers or crew members in scheduled domestic air transport accidents in 1970, the first fatality-free year in aviation. Preliminary figures indicate that general aviation deaths decreased to 1,270 in 1970 from 1,495 in 1969.

Home Accidents

Killed—27,000, unchanged from 1969.

Injured—4,100,000.

Cost—$1,800,000,000.

Deaths decreased in the 0-4-year and over-75-year age groups; increases occurred in all other age groups.

There were decreases in deaths from mechanical suffocation and falls; no change in poisoning by gas; and increases in poisoning by solids and liquids, firearms and fires, burns.

Fire Losses

The value of property destroyed by fires in 1970 was about $2,250,000,000, or 15 per cent more than in 1969.

The Eighth Revision of the International List of Diseases and Causes of Death was put into effect during 1968. This is the official list used by vital statisticians to classify deaths. Because figures for 1968 and 1969 have not yet been published by the national vital statistics agency it is not known just how much the changes in the list will influence the accidental death totals, but it is likely that the final overall figures may be lower than the estimates.

Figure 1. Reproduced from *Traffic Safety*, March 1971 with permission of National Safety Council.

Accidental Deaths in the United States
1959-1969

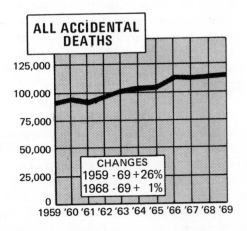

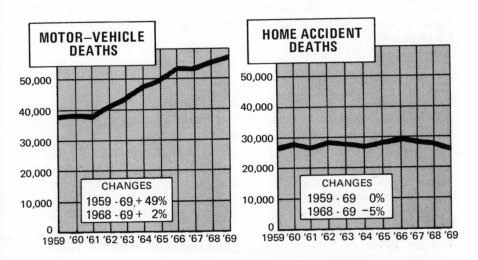

Figure 2. Reproduced from *Accident Facts 1970, Preliminary Condensed Edition, February 1970* with permission from the National Safety Council.

400,000 or more of these patients now have some degree of permanent impairment. Approximately one out of every four American people suffers from an accident of some degree each year and approximately one out of every eight beds in general hospitals in the United States is occupied by an accident victim. The total number of non-disabling injuries treated at home, in doctors' offices, and in out-patient clinics or emergency departments is unknown.

Each year it is estimated that over 500,000,000 days of restricted activity are the result of accidental injury, or nearly 20 percent of the restricted activity from all medical causes. Short-term conditions of restricted activity due to accidental injury exceed even the common cold. Injury admissions are estimated to result in the utilization of over 22,000,000 hospital bed days which is the leading cause of all bed day utilization in general hospitals. These figures are significantly higher than those for 1963.

The tangible economic loss expressed as costs and expenses from accidents is estimated by the National Safety Council to be over $22,000,000,000 a year. Part of this loss is visible, but much of it is not apparent except to the victims, their families, medical and hospital personnel, lawyers, employers, the courts, insurance companies, and workmen's compensation commissions.

Accidents cause impairment, disability, hospitalization, loss of days from work or school, and human grief for which we have no statistics. Therefore, the cost to the nation, while it includes the cost of hospitalization and resultant disability, cannot include the loss of working capacity and the ability to enjoy life (Figure 3).

Historical Context

The prominence of death from accidents is being recognized as a phenomenon of the twentieth century. In 1900, accidents ranked fourth as a cause of total deaths. However, during the intervening 40 years, while deaths from accidents have remained between 40 and 60 per 100,000 population, there has been a steady drop in the death rate from other major causes so that in the period from 1935 to 1940 accidents *for the first time* exceeded all other causes of death in the ages one through thirty-four years.

While the accidental death rates per 100,000 population or per 100 million miles of vehicular travel have decreased during this time, the increase in population and automobiles has resulted in an increase in the absolute death rate in all categories. Among the major causes of accidental death and disability, the automobile is unsurpassed. As noted in the *New York Times* (4/5/70), the level of mortality in accidents is closely related to the use of motor vehicles. Ever increasing horsepower coupled with an unchanging degree of human error has exceeded the rate of our willingness or ability to incorporate safety features into

Costs of accidents in 1970

The accidents in which the deaths and injuries occurred, together with noninjury motor-vehicle accidents and fires, cost the nation in 1970, at least

$27,000,000,000

THESE COSTS INCLUDE:

Wage losses due to temporary inability to work, lower wages after returning to work due to permanent impairment, present value of future earnings lost by those totally incapacitated or killed $7,200,000,000

Medical fees, hospital expenses $2,900,000,000

Insurance administrative and claim settlement costs (claims are not identified separately but losses for which claim payments are made are included in other items in this table — see note below) $5,900,000,000

Property damage in motor-vehicle accidents $4,700,000,000

Property destroyed by fire $2,263,000,000

Money value of time lost by workers other than those with disabling injuries, who are directly or indirectly involved in accidents $4,000,000,000

NOTES ON CERTAIN ACCIDENT COSTS

There are alternative ways of identifying certain costs of accidents. The items in the table above represent one of the ways. All measurable costs have been included, and none have been included twice. See comments below under insurance costs.

Wage losses. Loss of productivity by injured or killed workers is a loss to the nation. Since, theoretically, a worker's contribution to the wealth of the nation is measured in terms of wages, then the sum total of wages lost due to accidents provides a measure of this lost productivity. For nonfatal injuries, actual wage losses are used for fatalities and permanently disabling injuries, the figure used is the present value of all future earnings lost.

Insurance administrative and claim settlement costs. This is the difference between premiums paid to insurance companies and claims paid by them; it is their cost of doing business and is a part of the accident cost total. *Claims* paid by insurance companies are not identified separately in the total. Since every claim is paid to a claimant for such losses as wages, medical and hospital expense, etc., losses for which claims are paid are already included in various items in the table.

Figure 3. Reproduced from *Accident Facts 1971* with permission from the National Safety Council.

our automobiles. The mortality for most serious diseases in the United States is stationary or decreasing. The mortality from vehicular injury is steadily increasing.

In 1970, deaths alone from auto accidents were 55,300 — nearly 50 percent of the total accidental deaths — and are estimated to have cost $11,300,000,000. This amounts to an increase by a factor of 29 times since 1910.

The tragedy of the high traffic death rate is that this trauma kills thousands who otherwise could expect to live long and productive lives. Thus, many more man-years are lost owing to trauma deaths than from deaths due to chronic diseases. It is estimated that since 1903 when the "horseless carriage" emerged on our roads, there have been more than 6,500,000 deaths from accidents in this country and over 1,600,000 of these involved motor vehicles.

The trend in accident death rates for children has been downward since 1900, but the proportion of absolute childhood deaths due to accidents has been increasing. In 1966, four out of every ten children who died in this country were victims of trauma. Injuries have been the leading cause of death in children for over ten years. The hospital morbidity and long-term sequelae of injury in children have greater medical and social significance than in adults. Haller has reported (5) that more than 100,000 children are permanently crippled in the United States each year by accidents and another 2,000,000 temporarily incapacitated by injury. This is in addition to approximately 13,000 deaths from accidents between the ages of one and fourteen years. With the increasing number of children in our population, the enormous rehabilitation program necessitated by these injuries will certainly have to increase in equal ratio.

People over 65 are the victims of three-quarters of all of the fatal falls of this country and of one-third of all the pedestrian deaths due to motor vehicles. Over 28,000 people over the age of 65 died of accidental injuries during 1968. Falls accounted for almost half of the injuries sustained by the elderly. Death rates from motor vehicle accidents to pedestrians are extremely high in elderly patients. Several reasons for this are thought to be the physical decline with age and the unpredictability of the elderly pedestrian.

REFERENCES

1. Iskrant, A.P., and Joliet, P.S. *Accidents and Homicide.* Cambridge, Mass.: Harvard University Press, 1968.
2. *Traffic Safety,* March *1970.* National Safety Council.
3. *Accident Facts 1970, Preliminary Condensed Edition,* February *1970.* National Safety Council.
4. *Accident Facts* 1969. National Safety Council.
5. Haller, J.A., Jr. "Problems in Children's Trauma." *J. Trauma* 10 (March 1970): 269.
6. "Accidental Death and Disability: The Neglected Disease of Modern

Society." National Academy of Sciences, National Research Council, September 1966.

7. "Training of Ambulance Personnel and Others Responsible for Emergency Care of the Sick and Injured at the Scene and During Transport." National Academy of Sciences, National Research Council, March 1968.

8. "Medical Requirements for Ambulance Design and Equipment." National Academy of Sciences, National Research Council, September 1968.

9. "Report of the Secretary's Advisory Committee on Traffic Safety." United States Department of Health, Education and Welfare, February 1968.

10. Von Wagoner, F.H. "Died in Hospital: A Three Year Study of Deaths Following Trauma." *J. Trauma* 1 (1961): 401-408.

11. Frey, C.F., Huelke, D.F., and Gikas, P.W. "Resuscitation and Survival in Motor Vehicle Accidents." *J. Trauma* 9 (1969): 292.

12. National Institute of General Medical Sciences. "Report: Conference on Trauma." Public Health Service publication no. 1565, February 1966.

Section II

Principles of First Aid

Surprising New Facts about First Aid

Jean Carper

Would you slap a choking person on the back? Or put iodine on wounds? Or cut the traditional X in case of snakebite? Or even use ointment on burns or a tourniquet to stop bleeding? Then your first aid is out of date. But it's not surprising, for many once-popular treatments have changed radically in the light of new medical knowledge.

Here, according to the experts, are nine first-aid measures that have fallen from medical favor, but are still widely used. Here, too, are the newest lifesaving procedures that everyone should know:

Old Way: If someone is bitten by a poisonous snake, immediately cut an X through the fang marks and suck out the venom.

New Way: This "woods surgery" may have saved many a life in pioneer days. Today, however, the X-cut is rarely necessary *if you can reach a hospital within an hour*, says Dr. Henry Parrish, professor at the University of Missouri and noted snakebite authority.

There's little need to panic over snakebite. The amazing fact is that two-thirds of all persons bitten by poisonous snakes in this country get so little poison in their systems that they will survive with no treatment at all! Even in potentially fatal cases, the vast majority of victims have plenty of time to reach a doctor for an injection of antivenin to counteract the poison. Snake venom spreads very slowly through the system, much like ink being absorbed into a blotter. And far from happening in the wilds, most snakebites occur so close to civilization that 65 percent of the victims show up at a hospital within one hour.

Instead of the cut-and-suck method, tie a constricting band around the limb about two inches above the bite. Don't cut off circulation; make the band just tight enough so you can still wedge a finger under it. Keep the victim as motionless as possible to retard the spread of venom. If medical help is more than an hour away, cut just through the skin and suck the wound only if symptoms of poisoning are apparent (swelling, pain, and redness around the puncture wounds). Contrary to popular belief, there is virtually no danger in taking venom into your mouth, and most snakes are non-poisonous.

Old Way: When a person is choking, slap him on the back to dislodge the obstruction.

New Way: Resist the impulse. A slap on the back, far from being harmless, is potentially deadly, medical specialists now tell us.

A choking fit is usually triggered by food or some other object lodging

Reprinted with permission from *Today's Health*, November 1966, Vol. 44, No. 11, pp. 20-23, published by the American Medical Association.

where it shouldn't be — in the voicebox at the entrance to the windpipe. To get rid of the object, the voicebox goes into violent muscle spasms. If the muscles are given time to relax, the person ordinarily coughs up the object.

But suppose you slap him on the back? This forces him to involuntarily take a gasp of air. Have someone slap you sharply between the shoulder blades and you'll see. The inrush of air through the voicebox may suck the object on down into the windpipe, possibly deep into the lungs.

Sometimes the foreign object slips into the windpipe, but only partially plugs it. In this situation, a slap on the back may induce the victim to cough the object back up against the narrower opening at the vocal cords, causing complete air blockage and asphyxiation.

The best first aid for choking is the least. "Do nothing momentarily," advises Dr. Paul G. Bunker, former vice president of the American Broncho-Esophagological Association. "Try to get the victim to relax and give the cough reflex — which is nature's built-in safeguard — time to work. The coughing will usually expel the object. Only if the person stops breathing and is obviously in danger of dying should you slap him on the back in a last-ditch effort to dislodge the object." Then hold him head down or lay him across something head down, and slap him hard between the shoulder blades. A small child can be up-ended.

Old Way: If a child is poisoned, give him the "universal antidote" — a potent lifesaver that you can buy at a pharmacy or mix up at home.

New Way: Although the so-called universal antidote received a flurry of publicity several years ago and is still recommended in nine important first-aid books, don't depend on it.

Theoretically it is supposed to counteract most types of poisons. The commercial version is made from tannic acid (to neutralize alkalies), magnesium oxide (to neutralize acids), and activated charcoal (to absorb poisons), and does have some value because of the charcoal's fantastic abilities to soak up certain poisons in the stomach. A chemist once swallowed a potentially lethal dose of arsenic trioxide, mixed with charcoal, and lived to write about it.

However, University of Arizona pharmacologists have just discovered that the absorption of poison is one-third greater with activated charcoal alone than with the "universal antidote." For some reason, the acid and magnesium oxide reduce the lifesaving powers of the charcoal in some instances.

Nothing good whatever can be said for the homemade "universal antidote" of burned toast (charcoal), tea (tannic acid), and milk of magnesia (alkali). It's one of those monumental mistakes that sounded good, but turned out to be worthless. "Pure myth," says Henry L. Verhulst, head of the U.S. Public Health Service's National Clearinghouse for Poison Control Centers. Tests reveal that charcoal from burned toast is not the type that absorbs poison.

Some health officials now urge parents to keep two antidotes on their shelves: plain activated charcoal, which you mix with water in case of poisoning, and syrup of ipecac, which produces vomiting. Both are available at pharmacies without prescription. Before using either, however, it's best to consult a doctor. Vomiting is exceedingly dangerous if the child has swallowed petroleum products (gasoline, lighter fluid) or strong corrosives (lye, drain cleaner). Also, charcoal is not effective against some poisons.

Old Way: When burned, cover the skin with ointment or a solution of baking soda.

New Way: "Avoid ointments, greases, and baking soda, especially on a burn bad enough to require medical treatment," says Dr. John A. Boswick, director of hand and burn surgery at Chicago's Cook County Hospital. Although they relieve pain by excluding air, these home remedies can be harmful. Doctors must always scrape them off, which delays treatment and can be excruciatingly painful. An unsterile grease or soda solution can contribute to infection. What's more, neither hastens healing.

Doctor Boswick and many colleagues recommend only one first-aid treatment for lesser burns: cold water. As American doctors have rediscovered in the last five years, cold water dramatically relieves pain, and there is suggestion that it reduces scarring and promotes healing of burned flesh. In one case, a California workman who was badly scalded by steam received ice compresses on all burned areas except a tiny patch of abdominal skin that was overlooked. The very next day all of the burned skin treated with ice water was completely healed, but the small neglected patch of skin blistered and did not heal for two weeks.

Doctors believe that cold water may be beneficial to all burns, but in the absence of conclusive evidence, they currently advocate its use on lesser burns only, covering under 10 percent of the body. In case of more extensive burns, your time is better spent getting to a hospital, they say.

Submerge the burned skin immediately (the sooner, the better the results) in *comfortably* cold water, usually under 70° F. Add ice to keep the water cold. On burned parts that can't be immersed, apply cloths soaked in ice water and change the cold packs constantly at first. Continue treatment until you can keep the burned part out of cold water without having pain recur.

Old Way: To stop serious bleeding, never touch the wound with your hand or unsterile material. Apply a tourniquet.

New Way: Thanks to antibiotics, the day that you dared not touch an open wound for fear of deadly infection has disappeared — and with it so has the vicious tourniquet. Today, we can use the direct approach: Simply put a cloth (sterile, if possible; there's no sense asking for infection) over the wound. If you don't have a clean cloth, use a wad of clean tissue, your bare hand or fingers. Then press hard. The pressure will squeeze the blood vessels against tissue, muscles, or bone, and will usually stop the flow if you press hard enough.

The tourniquet these days is viewed with absolute horror. Everyone, including the armed forces and the American Red Cross, has banned its use except in rare life-and-death emergencies where bleeding can't be controlled any other way, as when a limb is so obviously mangled that it probably will be lost.

Properly applied, a tourniquet cuts off all blood circulation to the limb with the eventual risk of tissue death (gangrene) and amputation. To prevent this, surgeons previously recommended loosening the tourniquet several times an hour to let blood flow through the limb. This practice, doctors discovered, lost more lives than it saved.

A sufficiently tight tourniquet stops the hemorrhage, but also means that the deep tissues, especially large masses of muscle, promptly asphyxiate and begin to die. Poisonous substances form in the asphyxiating limb and when the tourniquet is loosened, these toxins get into the patient's circulation and cause a condition called "tourniquet shock." This sometimes deepens steadily until the patient dies.

If it has been necessary to apply a tourniquet so tight that it stops circulation, and if it has maintained this condition for more than a few minutes, it should be removed only by a physician prepared to combat the ensuing shock. The modern dictum: "Apply a tourniquet only if you are willing to sacrifice the limb" makes irrefutable scientific sense.

Old Way: To kill germs on wounds, apply an antiseptic such as iodine, and never use soap and water.

New Way: Medical men now caution: Don't use antiseptics; wash out a wound with gauze or cotton soaked in soap and water.

Some antiseptics aren't as effective as soap and water in preventing wound infections and they have harmful side effects. For example, if iodine is kept around the house for any length of time, the alcohol will evaporate. When used, it can destroy living tissue around the wound and retard healing.

Soap and water, on the other hand, doesn't injure tissue, does kill some germs, and provides a marvelous flushing action that washes away armies of bacteria. For example, soap and water has proved incredibly effective in floating away the rabies virus from animal-bite wounds. Recent experiments with animals at New York State's Department of Health laboratories show that when rabies-infected wounds go untreated, there's only a 10 percent chance of survival. But scrubbing and flushing the infected wounds with soap and water increases the survival odds *nine times*, to an astounding 90 percent.

Old Way: You see a swimmer dive in and strike his head; you must quickly get him out of the water to prevent drowning.

New Way: Let him float in the water; never hurriedly drag him out. From a four-year study of diving injuries in New Jersey, Dr. Richard Rado estimates that 750 divers suffer broken necks yearly in the United States, and 500 of them wind up paralyzed — often because a bystander's impulse is to "get them out."

Consider these two cases: After a 12-year-old girl in an Eastern city broke her neck during a shallow dive in a backyard pool, her panicked father dragged her down a four-foot ledge and carried her into the house with her head dangling. That child today is paralyzed from the neck down.

In the same city, a young man struck his head in a public pool and was temporarily paralyzed. Still conscious, he begged bystanders to take him out. Instead, a friend jumped in and supported the victim floating on his back until ambulance personnel arrived and lifted him out on a spine board. Orthopedic surgeons said this diver had the worst neck fracture they had seen. Yet he quickly recovered without a trace of paralysis, solely because he was carefully taken from the water with no yanking or twisting of his neck.

It is imperative after any diving accident to protect the neck. Often, a neck vertebra has shattered, allowing bone splinters to project perilously close to the spinal cord, which is finger-thick and fragile as stiff gelatin. One wrench of the neck can drive a bone sliver into the soft spinal cord. The inevitable result is lifelong paralysis; for once damaged, the cord, being nerve tissue, will never heal.

The proper action is clear: Always help an injured diver stay afloat; the water is an excellent splint, and you can administer mouth-to-mouth resuscitation while he's in the water if necessary. Remove him only on a rigid stretcher — a spine board, surf board, door, wooden plank — anything that will keep his head absolutely level with his body.

Old Way: Rub frostbite with snow or massage the frozen limb and thaw it very slowly in cold water.

New Way: Whatever you do, avoid both rubbing and cold. As one doctor says: "Treating a cold injury with cold makes about as much sense as treating a burned foot by putting it in an oven." Nevertheless, medical men for years advised packing a frozen foot in snow or dunking it in cold water because such therapy accomplished a slow-thaw. And a slow-thaw, they believed, prevented tissue damage.

Navy experiments and recent cases in Alaska now prove the opposite: Deeply frozen limbs thawed very slowly in snow, cold water, or even at room temperature must be amputated most often, while those thawed faster in warm water baths are most often saved. One Alaskan surgeon, after using the warm water thaw, made only one frostbite amputation in five years: a big toe.

Rubbing frostbite, especially with rough-textured snow granules is absolutely verboten. Such massaging can rupture the skin cells and interfere with the circulation of blood. This may result in infection, gangrene, and even necessitate amputation. Gentle treatment of thawing tissue is so critical that in hospitals the frozen part is often suspended or packed in soft absorbent material so it can't even touch bed sheets.

To thaw frostbitten tissue the new fast way, immerse it in warm water, comfortable to the normal unfrozen hand, but not over 104° F. As soon as a flush extends to the tips of fingers and toes, the limb is thawed and you should remove it immediately. On frozen ears and noses, apply cloths soaked in warm water. Handle the frostbitten part with the utmost care and always see a doctor.

Old Way: Get an accident victim to a hospital with all possible speed. Every minute saved is a life-and-death matter.

New Way: Stifle the urge for precipitate action. Hastily moving an injured person can be disastrous. Recently, a woman in New England held off a whole crowd of angry onlookers who wanted to pick up a youngster struck down by a car and rush him to a hospital. She insisted that they wait for an ambulance — and fortunately, too, for the boy had spinal damage and moving him could have made him a lifelong cripple.

It's equally risky to drag victims from automobile crashes, for they too often have spinal injuries. Less-than-tender treatment can also cause a broken rib to puncture a lung, or increase hemorrhaging, or produce fatal shock. The American College of Surgeons urges you not to move an injured person — and that includes those who have fallen — unless the victim is exposed to greater dangers, such as fire or drowning. Give first aid where he lies and wait for experienced ambulance personnel to do the moving.

You rarely need to worry about racing a person to a hospital if adequate care has been provided at the accident site. It has been proved that in most accident cases, the few minutes gained do not make a whit of difference in whether the victim lives or dies. Only in poisoning are minutes crucial.

In fact, a high-speed, jostling, weaving ride through traffic often increases physical shock, say doctors. And ironically, many persons have been killed in accidents while racing at breakneck speed to consult a doctor about minor injuries.

Says Dr. Preston Wade, chairman of the board of regents of the American College of Surgeons: "Good first aid and driving within speed limits invariably do more to save an injured person's life than a high-speed race to the hospital."

What's Wrong with First Aid?

Preston A. Wade, M.D.

The increasing number of accident victims has created a serious problem for hospitals and the medical profession throughout the country.

Many other types of serious medical problems can be handled in specific centers when the delay caused by transportation is of no importance. In the treatment of the accident victim, however, every case is an emergency and needs treatment at or near the site of the accident. Therefore, all communities, small or large, and all hospitals in every area are receiving an increasing number of these patients, and national organizations such as the American Society for the Surgery or Trauma and the American College of Surgeons have recognized the importance of the problem and are attempting to improve the care of the accident victim.

Two Important Phases

The two important phases in the treatment of an injured person are the immediate care and the definitive care. The responsibility for the definitive care is usually assumed by an experienced surgeon in a hospital where proper assistance and equipment is available. This phase of the treatment is purely one for the medical profession and is receiving increasing attention from medical schools and from the medical profession as a whole.

The most important phase in treatment is the immediate care of the patient because the end result in many of the injured cases depends entirely upon the early treatment.

First aid at the scene of the accident is usually administered by a layman, and in many instances by an untrained person who has no knowledge of first aid principles. Transportation of the injured is in most instances afforded by a passer-by, ignorant of the proper methods of transportation, and the treatment afforded the patient in the accident room in many hospitals across the nation leaves much to be desired.

Simple, Sensible, Practical

The medical profession assumes a considerable share of responsibility in the education of the lay public in first aid matters, even more responsibility for the improvement in the transportation of the injured, and must assume the entire responsibility for the quality of the care rendered the injured person in the accident rooms of the hospitals.

The need for instruction to the lay public in first aid principles has been

Reprinted with permission from *Traffic Safety*, January 1959, Vol. 59, No. 1, pp. 8-10.

recognized for years, and great strides have been made by the Red Cross, in particular, in transmitting this information to the public. It is, however, necessary to emphasize continually to the public the necessity for continual instruction in first aid, not only for the isolated accident case but because of the danger of disasters or even atomic war. Those who are charged with the responsibility of teaching first aid should make a reasonable effort to see that the principles outlined are simple, sensible, and practical.

Fortunately, most of the first aid handbooks are deleting some of the ridiculous exercises so laboriously studied by the first aid groups in World War II — such as the absurd instruction concerning pressure point control of hemorrhage, and the emphasis on the tourniquet for bleeding limb, as well as the ridiculous instructions about giving an injured patient a drink of water or a stimulant.

There are some very simple steps the first aid student should know. There are certain urgent requirements in the immediate care of the traumatized patient, and there is a priority of procedure.

First: Open Air Way — The patient must have unrestricted respiration in order to survive. The interference with this normal breathing is usually the result of inhaled blood, mucus, or vomitus, and the first step is to remove this material from the mouth and the pharynx. Often, a crushing injury of the face or an injury to the lower jaws will so disturb the architecture of the mouth as to allow the tongue to drop backwards over the airway and cause interference with respiration.

A simple means of inserting a safety pin through the tongue and pulling the tongue forward and tying it to the clothing, if necessary, to allow the patient to continue to breathe is something that everyone should know. An open sucking wound of the chest should immediately be covered with a pressure dressing. This can be done by an untrained individual and is often a lifesaving measure.

Second: Control of Hemorrhage — So much misinformation has been published about the control of hemorrhage that it is necessary to reemphasize some of the general principles of its control. A pressure dressing is the proper method to stop hemorrhage. The pressure dressing is applied directly over the bleeding area and held in place by firm, but not tight, bandaging. The dressing may be applied by means of strips of clothing or other cloth.

A tourniquet should never be applied to a bleeding limb. This is something the layman refuses to believe, and his ignorance of the proper method of treatment is partly the fault of the medical profession in not insisting on this fact being publicized more frequently. Too often the newspapers give credit for the saving of a limb or a life to the application of a tourniquet. Rarely has a tourniquet ever saved a limb, but in many instances it has caused the loss of a limb or a life.

Sir Reginald Watson-Jones, the famous English surgeon, has advocated that the tourniquet be removed from all first aid kits so that the ignorant may not be tempted to use it. Even when a limb is completely severed, the blood vessel which is severed will, by reason of its spasm, close itself to a great extent, and fatal hemorrhage will not occur. It is only in the case of a partially torn vessel that a tourniquet would ever be necessary, and since a fatal hemorrhage would occur in a few moments, the tourniquet must be applied immediately.

Tourniquets applied too loosely will cause increased venous bleeding, if applied too tightly will cause damage to nerves and blood vessels, and if left too long may result in gangrene of a limb. Tourniquets left on for a prolonged period usually result in death.

There is very little that can be done to treat shock at the roadside, but a great deal can be done to prevent it or to lessen its severity. Care in the handling of the patient, stoppage of hemorrhage, splinting of the fracture, and care in transportation are the most essential factors in the treatment of shock. The patient should be covered, but no external heat should be applied. He should not be given stimulants, and he should not be given morphine, unless it is indicated for severe pain. The patient in shock is usually not in pain, and the indiscriminate use of morphine for shock is recognized as poor treatment.

Fourth: Splinting of Fractures — All fractures or limbs suspected of being fractured should be splinted immediately. The dictum of the Fracture Committee of the American College of Surgeons, "splint 'em where they lie," is one that should be taught to all first aid students.

The splints can be applied simply and easily by binding the upper extremity to the body using boards or magazines as splints for the forearms and binding the legs together for fractures of the thigh if Thomas splints or other board splints are not available for traction on the limb.

To attempt to teach the lay public intricate hitches for traction of the lower extremity is indeed a mistake. A simple board splint two feet longer than the leg may be laid along the side of the leg and its end inserted into the fold of an encircling sling at the groin. A bandage around the ankle is tied around the opposite end of the board. This affords, by means of a Spanish windlass, a gentle traction which will help in preventing shock as a result of a fractured thigh. Pillows and boards make excellent splints for legs and knees and are simply applied.

Fifth: Transportation of the Injured — So far in our discussion we have emphasized care in handling of the patient, and this is also most important in transportation, but most often overlooked. The natural inclination of the bystander is to consider speed the most important factor, when as a matter of fact it may be very harmful.

The patient should be properly splinted and should be transported on a flat board, stretcher, or litter if possible. If none of these are available at the scene of the accident, the patient must be transported as gently as possible and with as little movement as possible. This may be done by means of a blanket or merely by the simple process of four people lifting the patient by holding his clothes, while a fifth person supports his head.

In any case, the patient should be transported as gently as possible and flat on his back in a straight position. The habit of lifting a patient by knees and shoulders, doubling up his spine, is apt to be harmful. He should not be sat up but should be laid out in the back seat of a car if an ambulance is not available.

It is also the general habit of the public and ambulances, unfortunately, to consider speed as an essential part of the transportation of the patient. The more carefully the patient is transported, the better. This holds true for ambulances as well as other vehicles. It is the responsibility of the medical profession to denounce the tradition of speed in transportation of the injured in ambulances. The speeding ambulance injures and kills more people than it saves. There is rarely an instance in which a few minutes more or less would make any difference to the patient, while there are many instances in which the patient, the driver, the doctor, and other innocent victims are injured or killed by the ridiculous speed at which ambulances are operated.

Slowly this fact is being accepted in many communities, and in the future local ordinances and state laws will insist that ambulances obey traffic laws just as any other vehicle. The thrill of the speed and the pleasure of special privilege is really the reason for the speed of most ambulance drivers. A study of the ambulance calls of Flint, Michigan, by Curry and Lyttle has shown that in not a single instance of ambulance calls was there any evidence that speed changed the outcome of the case.

Sixth: Accident Room Care – The American College of Surgeons recognizes the fact that accident room care in this country can be improved and is, therefore, initiating at the Cornell University Medical College a study of the care of the injured in accidents throughout the country. This study has just been begun, but when it is completed, it is hoped that a set of minimum standards may be established which will help hospitals to satisfy what will be considered requirements necessary for the number of injured that may be expected in a given area.

It has long been the attitude of many hospitals that an accident victim deserved only such attention as may be available at the time of his admission to the hospital. Since the injury is an act of God, the hospital does not feel that it should necessarily be prepared at all times to take care of these accidents. The College of Surgeons would like to dispel this attitude and to emphasize that every hospital has a responsibility in·being prepared for not only the isolated accident victim but for a considerable number of injured that might appear as a result of a catastrophe.

Deserve Expert Care

In many instances the first person to see the patient in the hospital is the most inexperienced member of the staff, and he often is charged with the responsibility of the early care of the injured patient. It is the duty of the hospital to see to it that a well-qualified member of the staff is assigned to each case and that he personally sees, examines and directs the treatment of the injured victim.

It is the duty of the hospital to see that the emergency room is supplied with the material necessary for a reasonable number of cases.

We might summarize what I consider to be the most important points I have tried to make by quoting an old-time upstate New York country practitioner whose son was a student of mine. He stopped me on graduation day and said something like this: "My son has come back with a lot of things he says you told him that seem tommyrot to me. He says you insist on no tourniquet for hemorrhage, no morphine for shock, and no speed for the ambulance and insist on the patient seeing the chief surgeon when he gets to the hospital. And on top of all this, he tells me that you say there's no such thing as a whiplash injury and that it's only a pain in the neck, and not only to the patient alone. If these things are true, I'll certainly have to change a lot of my old ideas." I certainly hope that he does.

Suddenly . . . You're Involved!

Carl J. Potthoff, M.D.

Of the estimated 91 million Americans who were licensed to drive in 1962, about 19 million were involved in motor vehicle accidents during that year. This is about one out of every five drivers, but since some were involved in more than one accident, the number may be closer to one out of six.

These statistics provide a clue to the number of reportable accidents in which a driver is involved during his lifetime. Assuming an operating lifetime as 50 years and a ratio of involved drivers to total drivers as one-fifth in each year, drivers, on the average, participate in about 10 motor vehicle accidents in a lifetime.

When an accident occurs, the driver suddenly comes under obligations. The stakes may be high, perhaps involving large sums of money, permanent cosmetic damage, physical and mental health, and sometimes death. An accident may be one of those key events in a driver's life that affects his future substantially.

The obligations extend to the beginning teen-age driver as well as to all others. Society invests the teen-ager with a mantle of adulthood when it issues him a driving license. Vehicle codes make no distinction in responsibilities of licensees according to age. Society clearly takes the position that the youthful driver has attained such stature that his decisions are wise even when he must deal with catastrophic accidents affecting life and limb.

The obligations placed upon involved drivers cannot be delegated, except sometimes in part, to others such as police officers at hand. Accident situations differ greatly; the problems differ, and sometimes there are no experienced people at hand.

Consider that virtually all vehicle operators drive on rural roads as well as on urban, where ambulance and medical services are quickly at hand and where they are not, where police may be summoned within reasonable time and where they cannot, at night as well as during daytime, in good weather as well as in bad.

It is unrealistic, therefore, to believe that you as an involved driver can look always to others. Sometimes you must take full charge, make the important decisions, and do what needs to be done. Always you have stipulated responsibilities.

The experience of physicians and attorneys shows that many involved drivers deal with their accident problems in ways that are contrary to law, to the welfare of injured persons, and to their own self-interests. The shortcomings

Reprinted from *Today's Health*, June 1964, Vol. 2, No. 6, pp. 27-29 and 65-66, published by the American Medical Association.

result mostly from ignorance — that is from failure to study beforehand what to do.

Because of such failure, we may, for example, not be alerted to the fact that an apparently insignificant accident can have a disastrous aftermath. It did not seem important to one driver that the fender of his automobile rubbed against that of another, and caused both automobiles to swerve sharply. But the resulting civil suit did seem important; it involved a claim for $200,000. The plaintiff alleged that a back injury was aggravated by the accident.

In another case, a driver failed to report an apparently insignificant accident to his insurance company. Some time later, when a civil suit was brought against him, he read the fine print in his personal liability insurance policy and learned that the insuring company could disclaim liability if a representative were not notified promptly after an accident. Many important insurance companies include a similar provision in their personal liability policies.

The steps to take if you are involved as a driver are: (1) comply with the law, (2) protect your self-interests, and (3) attend to injured persons. These three steps interweave and overlap.

Since legal obligations vary in the different jurisdictions, every driver should study his local traffic code. He should learn the rules of the road and what to do if involved in an accident. Are you, for example, required to stop before entering a public road from your private, home driveway? Are you under legal risk if you park farther from a curb than the law stipulates and an oncoming car strikes your protruding vehicle? Just what does your local law say regarding aid to the injured?

In general, local codes follow fairly closely the Uniform Vehicle Code. The stipulations of the 1962 revision of this Code are outlined here for instances in which there is property damage, or injury or death to any person. In such cases, if you are the driver, you have the following obligations:

1. Stop your vehicle immediately at the scene or as close thereto as possible, and remain at the scene until you have complied with the on-the-scene requirements. Such stop should be made without obstructing traffic more than is necessary.

2. You must give your name and address and the registration number of the vehicle you are driving to any injured person, other involved drivers, any occupant, or any person attending other involved vehicles, to persons attending damaged property, and to any police officer who is at the scene or who is investigating the accident. The Code also states that upon request and if available you must exhibit your driver's license or permit to drive to any of these people. Most or all state and local codes require that you must have your license or permit with you whenever you drive.

3. If no police officer is present and if none of the specified people are in condition to receive the information to which they are entitled, you must (after

fulfilling the other immediate requirements) forthwith report the accident to the nearest office of a duly authorized police authority and submit there the required information.

4. The Code states that if there has been injury or death as a result of the accident, or property damage estimated to be at least $25, $50, or $100, depending upon provisions of the local code, the driver of an involved vehicle must give notice of the accident to the nearest police authority by the quickest means of communication. Presumably, this stipulation would be regarded as fulfilled if a police officer obtains the information on the scene. If the driver is physically incapable of making this report, any other occupant of the vehicle must make the report or have it made.

5. If the vehicle you are driving collides with and damages an unattended vehicle or other property, you are required to stop, and locate and notify the operator or owner of the other vehicle or property, giving your name and address and that of the owner, if different, of the vehicle you are driving. The Code further states that if an unattended vehicle is damaged you should attach securely in a conspicuous place in or on the vehicle a written notice giving the name and address of the driver and owner of the vehicle doing the striking. Presumably this attached notice would suffice for the on-the-scene notification requirements if the owner or attendant cannot be located at the time.

6. The Uniform Vehicle Code also requires that a written report of certain accidents be made. Depending upon the provisions of the state and local codes, it states that a written report must be made within five or 10 days in case of injury or death or in case of property damage estimated to be at least $25, $50, or $100. This report is not required of people physically incapable during the period of incapacity, but if another person is the vehicle owner he must make the report. Except in certain particulars, such as identity of drivers and owners and the time and place of the accident, the information contained in this report is confidential, according to the Code.

7. The driver must render "reasonable assistance" to any person injured in the accident, "including the carrying, or the making of arrangements for carrying, of such person to a physician, surgeon, or hospital for medical or surgical treatment if it is apparent that such treatment is necessary, or if such carrying is requested by the injured person."

You protect your self-interest to some extent — but not completely — when you comply with the provisions of the law of the legal jurisdiction wherein the accident occurred. Additional steps commonly are advisable, for you may face civil suit later and you may have injuries that are manifest at once or become evident later. It is worth noting that court decisions are based upon evidence that is actually presented.

Here are five important points you should be aware of:

1. Warn oncoming traffic if there is a chance that a superimposed accident

may occur. How you warn depends upon circumstances. In urgent cases, you perhaps can send people in one or both directions to wave down traffic. You can place flares or other warning signals, taking care that they are sufficiently far away to give oncoming drivers ample time to stop. Ordinarily, such devices should be placed at least 100 yards away, and perhaps more than one should be placed in each direction. At night, have one or more automobiles drive upon the highway shoulder so that the lights will shine upon the accident scene. If you remove obstructing vehicles or other objects from the highway, make a written record of precisely where they were before removal.

2. Obtain and record information that may be useful in case of civil or criminal action, and for purposes of making out reports to police and insurance agents. Since this information is exceedingly important, it is advisable that you prepare yourself against the possibility of involvement in an accident by obtaining and studying the accident report forms of the local police authority and of your insurance company. All such forms are similar, at least roughly, and will guide you well concerning what information to obtain. You should always have a notebook and writing instrument in your vehicle.

Obtain and record information concerning precisely how the accident happened. Record the exact time and location, and the weather and road conditions. Record the positions of the vehicles after the accident and the evidences of skid marks, stepping off or otherwise measuring distances as seems indicated. Both diagrams and photographs of the accident scene may prove helpful to you later.

Be sure to obtain from the other driver the same information that you are required to give him under the vehicle code. Observe all involved people for evidences of injury or of lack of such evidence. For example, where had each occupant been sitting in the vehicle, what happened to each at the moment of impact, did they complain later, did they walk about, were they unconscious for a time, and what comments did they make? In emergency medical work we sometimes observe that drivers fail to ascertain even the license number of the other involved vehicle, the name of the driver, or whether the driver was the owner of the vehicle.

Obtain the names and addresses of all involved people, not only those of the driver and of witnesses. Forthright effort to get this important information concerning witnesses is advisable, because such people may promptly leave the scene.

3. Attorneys caution against making statements at the scene that directly or by inference constitute admission of having been at fault in the causation of the accident. The involved driver is likely to be so excited as to make rash, ill-considered remarks that are detrimental and unfair to himself. Attorneys also caution against making payments, even token payments, at the time, for thereby an admission of some fault may be implied. Except perhaps in clearly insignifi-

cant instances, it is highly advisable to consult an attorney, placing in his hands your legal problems and any responsibility regarding statements.

4. Have a medical checkup if there is any chance you are injured. The time lapse before you see your doctor may later be very important. The symptoms and signs of injury are often overlooked in the excitement of an accident. You should also urge all other people involved in the accident to see a doctor if there is any possibility that they have been injured.

5. Promptly notify the company or companies with which you have liability and collision insurance. Failure to make a prompt report may void your insurance policy.

The requirement to render reasonable assistance to injured victims applies to drivers whether or not they were at fault in causing the accident. Occasionally there is need to act quickly in rescuing a person or in giving first aid, but in the large majority of instances haste is not indicated. You may feel you have to hurry, and that you should make compromises from what is best because the victim is unconscious or seems near death, or because weather is inclement, or bystanders urge haste, or you have other things to do. Nevertheless, recalling that the stakes are high, take the time needed to assure good first aid, for thereby you protect both the victim and your own self-interests.

The likelihood of giving improper immediate care is greatest perhaps in case of an accident at night on a rural highway. Too often, involved drivers seem unwilling to walk some distances to a farmhouse or other site to summon expert help or to obtain suitable supplies and equipment. And so haste takes over; the victim's injured limb is not splinted; his extremity and perhaps his internal organs are damaged further when he is carried quickly to a vehicle, and he is transported sitting up in a passenger automobile.

The Uniform Vehicle Code makes no requirement regarding driver education in first aid. Nevertheless, the assistance given to an injured person should reflect, as a minimum, ordinary prudence and common sense, and be confined to what seems necessary as immediate first aid.

1. In a substantially large share of accident situations, the advisable course is to leave the severely injured people where they are, and summon an ambulance or physician to the scene. The arrangements can usually be planned with the victim or those accompanying him. If police are at hand, they will be of much assistance. Seriously injured persons should lie down. They may need covering. Ordinarily, blankets should not be slipped beneath a victim if an ambulance will arrive shortly, because the maneuver might cause additional damage. But if there is likely to be considerable delay under inclement weather conditions, the attempt should be made, using utmost care.

2. Occasionally a body part is subjected to the heavy, overlying weight of the vehicle. It may be possible with the aid of bystanders to relieve the victim,

perhaps using one or more automobile jacks or the lever action of poles. Great care for the safety of the rescuers and the victim should be exercised in the procedure.

3. Ordinarily, the only urgent first aid that may be needed is attention to severe bleeding and to respiratory difficulty. Bleeding from the body surface should be controlled by pressure with a pad of cloth, the cleaner the better, directly upon the wound. A snug bandage should be placed over the pad. The pad should not be removed when saturated with blood; instead, additional padding should be applied over the original one. Tourniquets seldom if ever are needed; they usually cause more damage than benefit.

If a victim has difficulty in breathing, bleeds from the mouth or nose, or vomits, carefully place him in a face-down position. He may be more comfortable if his chest is elevated somewhat by placing a coat or the like beneath it.

4. Most participants in accidents remain able to exercise their own judgment regarding what immediate attention they desire from you. If you think the course they propose to take is in error, the best you can do ordinarily is to present your suggestions. In situations where you have responsibility for making the decisions, the questions to be resolved include these: Should the person have medical attention? Should he be transported lying down? Should any extremities be immobilized? Examination at the scene is inadequate at best, and commonly not highly informative to a non-medical person, but the problems can be resolved intelligently. If a person is comatose, he clearly needs transportation in the lying-down position. If he is conscious, he can tell you where he has pain or discomfort, and whether he suspects injury to any extremity.

Perhaps you can make some observations cautiously, even upon strangers if they consent, such as of the upper extremity or the leg. A basic precept is to play the safe side when in doubt as to whether you should call an ambulance, transport in the lying-down position, or immobilize all extremities. Be particularly cautious when dealing with a person who has "blacked out" even momentarily or wishes to sit by for a time, any elderly person, child, or person under the influence of alcohol.

Fractures may cause little or no pain when kept immobile, and sometimes very little despite appreciable motion of distal parts such as fingers. Consider the chance of hip fracture, especially in an elderly person, despite absence of any evidence except that he is reluctant to stand. Immobilize what you surmise are sprained extremity parts. These problems show the advisability of summoning expert help whenever injuries conceivably may be serious.

5. If an injured person must be moved, the body parts should be kept immobile in relationship to each other — that is, no part should bend, twist, dangle, or come under strain. We cannot likely maintain such immobility,

preventing strain, pressure, and movement involving torn internal organs such as the liver and spleen, lacerated muscles, and fractured bones, if we move victims in the sitting-up position or permit them to walk.

Whether the transfer be only a few feet or many miles, whether by carry or by vehicle, the use of a stretcher, one that does not sag lengthwise in the middle, should be considered. Sometimes it is feasible to use a firm frame or a cot as an alternative. Thereby we maintain immobilization sufficiently well in virtually all cases except those involving fractures of the neck vertebrae and of long bones of the extremities.

Splints are used in case of suspected fractures of these extremity bones. There are standard ways to apply splints, but the basically important point to remember is this: Keep the broken bones and the adjacent joints immobile. Through muscle action, motion at adjacent joints affects the broken bones. Use one splint or, if necessary to the basic purpose, two on opposite sides. Use splints that are long enough to immobilize the affecting joints. For example, if a shinbone is possibly broken, a splint that extends from the heel to only just above the knee will not adequately immobilize the knee.

Limbs usually must be straightened if a splint is to be applied; but if there is marked pain at a joint such as the knee or elbow during the attempt, try to devise a means of immobilization with the joint bent as you find it. Avoid using unwieldly, ineffective improvisations. "Splint them where they lie" if possible. Splint even though you only suspect a fracture.

Fracture or dislocation of a neck vertebra is of utmost importance because the spinal cord may be affected. Injury to the cord may be manifest by weakness or paralysis of an extremity, or by numbness or a tingling feeling along a shoulder or arm. Improper transportation may result in death immediately or increase the chance of permanent paralysis. Therefore, if the injury is suspected, summon medical help. If rescue from imminent danger is absolutely necessary, manually immobilize the extended head, not permitting it to flex forward or sideways, and perhaps exert a little traction away from the body while others move the person.

6. If a seriously injured person must be moved, the safest course for both the welfare of the victim and your own self-interest as an involved driver is to obtain the services of experts. Occasionally, despite the inherent risks, the clearly sensible course may require that you take the responsibility and direct the procedure. You can markedly lessen the risks if you transport the person in the lying-down position, usually upon his back unless he vomits or has respiratory difficulty when supine, and if you provide a gentle rather than a speedy and punishing ride.

Transportation, however, embraces not only vehicular transfer but also moving the person a short distance, such as from a roadway or ditch, loading him upon a vehicle, and extricating him from his own vehicle. The danger in these short-distance transfers has not been emphasized sufficiently; it may be much greater than during vehicular transportation.

To illustrate the method for lifting and depositing a victim, let us assume that several persons are available to help carry the injured person. Two, or preferably three, should position themselves at one side of the victim, and the other carrier on the opposite side. One carrier should act as leader, stating precisely how the maneuver is to be executed and what his signals will be. The carriers should then kneel, each on the knee that is nearest the victim's feet, and slide their hands underneath in such position that they can support the head, trunk, and lower extremities in a straight line. At a signal, they raise the person to their knees, pause a moment, and then at another signal stand erect. When depositing the person, they first lower him to the knees and then to the ground.

It is possible that two persons of adequate strength can carry a badly injured victim safely even though they are inexperienced and do not use a stretcher. The degree of risk depends on the nature of the injuries. If an attempt is made, the two should place themselves on the same side of the victim. Should they face each other instead, one at the head end to support the head and shoulders, and the other at the lower extremities to support them, the patient is subject to grave danger because his spine and trunk become flexed when he is lifted, the internal organs are compressed, and the spine and spinal cord, if injured, may be damaged further.

There is no routine way to extricate victims from vehicles; the best method must be devised at the scene. Usually it is advisable to survey the situation first, ascertaining if possible what body parts are injured. If a fracture of an extremity bone is suspected, the extremity should be splinted before moving the person.

The strategic positioning of assistants is of much importance. Even though a lower extremity is splinted, it may be advisable to delegate to one person the task of supporting the extremity. He should place his hands underneath, one on each side of the fracture site, devoting himself to the task while others carry the principal weight of the body. Proceeding slowly and cautiously, avoiding torsion and flexion of the trunk, the carriers should be able to avoid causing additional injury.

Although the first aid information given here embraces the principal theoretical considerations, it does not constitute an adequate course in the subject. The benefits of taking a first aid course that includes both theory and practice should appeal to any person who foresees a lifetime of risk at the wheel.

The Vehicle Accident—Multiple Injuries

Keith John Karren, M.S.

A familiar sight and sound in America is the flashing red of an ambulance as it wails its way to a scene of mangled steel and bodies. More than one and a half million people have been killed in the U.S. since 1900, and each year there are over 10 million disabling injuries resulting from accidents. These tragic statistics have a definite message to people training in first aid procedures. Some 20,000 lives might be saved annually in the U.S. if the victims received better-trained attention at the accident scene and on the way to the hospital.

Most of those injured in a traumatic vehicle accident will experience multiple injuries. It is the multiple injury victim who will suffer the most from an uninformed or unwise samaritan who does not know what to do or how to do it. He may not know which priorities come first or how to protect the victim from further injury.

Approach to the Accident Scene

The early first aid begins with your approach to the accident scene. Don't stop your car in an obstructive place but drive slowly past if possible and then pull off the road. The ambulance, upon arrival, will then have a clear passage to the victims. If there are other people present and wondering what to do, quickly send one to call for an ambulance, police, and a wrecker truck. Give instructions to others to direct traffic at each approach by stopping all traffic or by operating a slow one-way system past the accident if it is safe. Appoint two others as "crowd marshals" to ask others to stand well back and off the road and not to smoke (cigarettes may ignite gasoline). Make sure the ignition is switched off on the accident vehicles.

Now it is time to treat the casualties, and a proper plan for dealing with priorities must be clear in your mind. Remember that erroneous first aid may be not only detrimental but even fatal. It is wiser not to administer doubtful and possibly harmful treatment.

Reassure the Victim

As you approach the victims, reassure them that they are going to be taken care of. This is especially important for the person who is making a big fuss. Dr. P.S. London, a surgeon in Birmingham Accident Hospital in England, said:

> "To most persons it is self-evident that an injury causes pain, the degree of which bears some relation to the degree of injury. In many cases the behavior of the injured person supports this belief. In fact, whereas mild injuries leave a person's anxieties and senses unimpaired, severe

injury dulls them to the point at which there may be not only no complaint of pain but little acknowledgement of pain. The person that makes a fuss is likely to be badly frightened rather than badly injured and will often respond well to firm reassurance." (1)

ORGAN-SYSTEM PRIORITIES IN THE
EMERGENCY FIRST AID OF THE MULTIPLE INJURY VICTIM

---

1. Adequate airway and heartbeat
2. Control bleeding and treat for shock
3. Rapid general survey
   a. Head injury
   b. Wounds of face, chest, and abdomen
   c. Internal injury
   d. Fractures and dislocations of extremities

Adequate Airway and Heartbeat

The most important priorities are the establishment and maintenance of adequate ventilation and adequate circulation. If the victim is breathing properly, if he's not bleeding to death, and if his circulatory system is not hampered by shock, all other body systems will function unless they are injured.

First, check for breathing by observing chest movement and coloring of the victim, especially the lips, ears, and fingernails. Simultaneously feel the pulse through the carotid artery on either side of the trachea in the neck. If you can detect no pulse or breathing, and the victim is beginning to exhibit a cyanotic or blue coloring, quickly administer mouth-to-mouth resuscitation with three good huffs of air and then give external cardiac massage for 30 seconds. Continue this process if you are alone or administer both complete processes if other first-aiders are present.

Many times in an auto accident the face structure is injured. In this situation, protect the airway from being blocked by bony fragments and have the victim sit up if he can and spit out the blood and secretions. If he can't sit up, have him lie on his side with his head to the side and inclined slightly downward so the victim's tongue will not fall back and strangle him. Keep the mandible forward and continue wiping the blood and secretions out of his mouth.

Control Bleeding

Next in priority is the controlling of any obvious hemorrhage. Direct pressure with the bare hand or a heavy gauze dressing is first applied. When the bleeding is controlled, apply a clean and, if possible, sterile dry dressing such as gauze and use a "conforming" bandage. Medication and cleansing are not required, but it is important to remove any loose foreign bodies and straighten any loose sections of skin.

Treat for Shock

Shock is defined as a "condition characterized by signs and symptoms that arise when the cardiac output is insufficient to fill the arterial tree with blood under sufficient pressure to provide organs and tissues with adequate blood flow." (7) This situation is closely associated with the trauma involved in a vehicle accident. Dr. James G. Chandler, in an article entitled "The Physiology and Treatment of Shock," explains three basic categories of shock.

1. Pump-failure shock, characterized by a primary failure of cardiac output.
2. Fluid-loss shock.
3. Peripheral resistance collapse shock, resulting either from a decrease in arterial tone or from an increase in capacitance of the venous capillary bed. (7)

The pump failure concerns the failure of the heart to pump the blood to the body. The fluid loss means the loss of blood and other body fluids, either by way of internal or external hemorrhage. The peripheral resistance collapse concerns the dilation or loss of resistance and consequent pressure in the circulatory system. Any one of these three circumstances results in a decreased amount of blood perfusing the body tissues and a decreased blood volume returning to the heart. This, of course, results in a decreased heart output and the deteriorating cycle continues to develop. The body tries to get blood to the brain, heart, and liver at all costs, with the kidneys being fourth in priority. This means that blood flow to the skin and especially the extremities is cut off. If this depression of circulation to vital organs deepens, tissues begin to die from anoxia.

Signs to look for in shock development include cold, clammy skin, mottled skin with a pallor complexion, cyanotic blue coloring of the extremities, weakness and faintness, eyes dull and vacant looking with dilated pupils, rapid and shallow breathing, weak irregular pulse, thirst, and restlessness.

Shock is to be feared in all accident situations, so either protect against or treat for shock by reassuring the victim, placing him in a horizontal position, and elevating the limbs. Have a blanket under and over the victim (after the general survey) to help keep body temperature normal. Give water or saline solution if you are sure there are no internal injuries.

General Survey

Head Injury.

Next, conduct a rapid general survey. You should begin at the head and proceed downward, observing the state of consciousness. Spinal fluid or blood coming from the nose or ears and the dilation or constriction of the victim's pupils are signs that may tell you of concussion or congestion of the brain. If the victim is unconscious and the other signs are positive, treat as for shock, except give nothing by mouth. You will have to obtain the services of a doctor immediately, being careful not to move the patient. If this isn't possible, finish the general survey, carrying out the necessary first aid, and then transport him on a stretcher lying flat on his back with as little movement as possible.

Wounds of Face, Chest, and Abdomen.

Wounds of face, chest, and abdomen receive special attention. Dressings on wounds of the face and jaw should be applied with an open airway in mind. Neck and chest wounds cause risks of air embolism and accumulation of air or gas in the pleural cavity, causing the lung on the injured side to collapse and also decreasing efficiency of the opposite lung. This type of wound can be recognized by a characteristic sucking sound or the victim breathing out bright red frothy blood. Quickly apply a bulky dressing to the wound as the victim breathes out and bind the dressing in place. The dressing will usually become airtight as the blood wets it.

Internal Injury.

Signs of internal injury should be constantly watched for in the case of a vehicle accident victim. These signs may include faintness, thirst, restlessness, vague feelings of great anxiety, and the other symptoms exhibited by shock. Early development of profound shock is a common sign of internal bleeding. Other signs to consider are coughed up blood that is bright red and frothy, bright red blood in the vomitus, or a stool streaked with red blood. If one or more of these signs indicate internal bleeding, keep the victim completely quiet in a slightly reclining position and give nothing by mouth. The bleeding will only be controlled by surgery, so a physician is imperative.

Fractures and Dislocations of Extremities.

The extremities should now be examined for fractures and dislocations which must be carefully splinted or immobilized. Guard against further injury. Notice whether the victim has the ability to move his extremities because this will give you an idea of spinal cord injury. If the victim can move his arms but not his legs, he may have injured the spinal cord in the thoracic area or lower. If he cannot move arms or legs he has probably injured the spinal cord in the cervical area. Any misalignment may cause permanent paralysis or even death. Regarding this, a noted American doctor said, ". . . most important is that the patient with a head injury has a cervical spine injury until it's proven otherwise." (2)

Extrication

Removing the victim from the wreckage is also a critical aspect of first aid. Dr. J.D. Farrington, an expert on accident care, said:

"The first point to remember in a rescue operation is that there's usually no hurry about extricating the victim." Speed would be essential only in the threat of fire or explosion. There is usually not much danger of these occurring.

If you suspect a spinal cord injury, keep the neck and spinal cord in constant alignment. Handle an unconscious victim as if he had a spinal cord injury. One of the finest techniques for doing this was developed by Dr. Farrington. He designed spine boards to splint the spine of the victim while he is still in the car. The first step is to apply a cervical collar in the case of a suspected neck injury. If one is not readily available, you can improvise by folding lengthwise some long thick 10-inch-wide bandages, placing these around the neck and fastening with safety pins. The short spine board is slid behind the sitting victim, who is then strapped to it. The long spine board is used to splint the victim who is laying down in the car. Specific instructions concerning the spine boards can be found in a number of first aid texts, particularly those written for rescue squads. The victim can now be slowly and safely removed by two first-aiders and placed on a litter or stretcher.

Transportation

By now we would hope an ambulance has arrived. If the situation requires you to provide the transportation to a medical facility, direct the evacuation of the victim and guard against further injury. Use a firm stretcher, either commercial or makeshift, in transporting the patient to a *suitable* vehicle (preferably a station wagon if available). An unconscious or semiconscious victim must be transported in the prone or semiprone position to reduce the risk of aspiration. Instruct the driver to be gentle, especially in curves and turns, and not to exceed the speed limit. "Haste in transportation of the sick and injured is unnecessary in about 98 per cent of the cases and will not noticeably alter the patient's course." (3)

The first-aider must use a systematic approach in the care of a multiple-injury victim. Some of the first aid procedures can be carried out simultaneously as one first-aider in charge gives directions. As a cautious, careful priority system is carried out, a victim who might otherwise have died is given another chance at life. Remember, it is good emergency first aid that saves lives!

REFERENCES

1. London, P.S. "Road Accidents and the Family Doctor." *British Medical Journal* 4(1969):285.

2. "The Multiple Injury Patient." *Ohio Medical Journal* 63(June 1967):789-801.
3. Young, Carl B. Jr. *First Aid for Emergency Crews.* Springfield, Ill.: Charles C. Thomas, 1970.
4. Currie, Donald V. "Early Management of the Critically Injured." *Canadian Medical Association* 95(22 October 1966):862-870.
5. Jolles, Keith E. "When the Accident Is All Yours." *Nursing Times* 64(26 January 1968):118-120.
6. "Extrication." *Emergency Medicine*, October 1969, pp. 35-43.
7. Chandler, James G. "The Physiology and Treatment of Shock." *RN*, June 1971, pp. 42-43, 76-81.

When to Leave the Scene of an Accident

The flooding Mississippi threatens a river town, and an army of teen-agers reinforce the levee.

Hurricane Betsy devastates the Gulf Coast, and entire communities turn out to feed the hungry and shelter the homeless.

A raging blizzard maroons families in New England, and hundreds of snow-mobilers plow to the rescue.

Natural disasters often bring out the best in people. So why is it that individual tragedies — traffic accidents in particular — often evoke one of man's worst traits, morbid curiosity?

A bad highway accident will attract crowds like desert carrion draws vultures. A state patrolman describes his arrival at an accident scene haunted by thrill-seekers:

"I saw the people watching. No one was helping. They were only standing, staring. They were completely absorbed by the spectacle of a grief-stricken husband trying to pump life back into the body of his dead wife. I wondered if these people were being entertained and why none of them had tried to help the poor man. Out of a crowd of people there usually are a few who will try to help."

As sad a commentary on human nature as that may be, it is not just the *attitude* of the accident gaper that is the problem. The chief difficulty is that curious, converging, standing, staring people *impede the work of handling an emergency and contribute to additional accidents.*

They impede rescue by getting in the way of professional people who are working at the scene. Perhaps they stop because they would like to be helpful but are really helpless, or maybe they're just fascinated by a grisly spectacle. But whatever their motives, the fact is that they can seriously impede rescue efforts when a life may be at stake.

Their randomly parked cars prevent emergency vehicles from getting close. In any collision there is danger of fire due to spilled gasoline, and fire engines, the slowest of all emergency vehicles, must get close when they do arrive.

In literally hundreds of cases, curiosity seekers have made a bad situation worse by causing other accidents at the scene — by braking suddenly, parking unsafely or walking around on the roadway. Many times — it happens almost daily — onlookers themselves are hurt at the misfortune they are gawking at. This happened recently to a motorist on Chicago's Eisenhower expressway who

Reprinted with permission from *Family Safety*, Vol. 29, No. 2, Summer 1970, pp. 8-9.

ran into a semi-trailer truck because he was staring at an accident instead of keeping his eyes on the road. Gapers can get surly — even unruly — when police officers attempt crowd control. They even throw rocks and bottles at policemen and firemen trying to clear the area for safety reasons.

But the morbidly curious are the hardest to understand. An officer reported this actual conversation at the scene of a fatal accident:

"Anybody killed, officer?"

"Yes."

"How many?"

"I don't know yet."

"I passed here a moment ago, and I told my wife that I bet somebody was killed. I told my wife that I was going to come back and find out."

The officer remembers that the man seemed pleased that he had guessed correctly and that he was smiling brightly as he looked over the scene in an apparent attempt to view a body.

Few people become hostile at an accident scene and few are truly morbid. But many — perhaps most — of us have the human trait of wanting to know what's going on. That's why we read newspapers and watch TV news shows. But curiosity must be overcome during the special circumstances of a highway accident as a matter of self-protection as well as for the safety of the many other people involved. An accident scene is a dangerous place for an onlooker to tarry. The sooner you can get away the safer you'll be.

Still, there may be times when you can be of genuine assistance — and perhaps save a life. It's important to judge when and know what to do. Too many variables make it difficult to set hard and fast rules, but experts agree on this general advice:

1. If you are first at the scene, park carefully, well away from traffic, and do what you can to help. If you're trained in first aid, treat the injured to the best of your ability. If you're sure you can do so without compounding injuries or if there is likelihood of fire, remove the victims as far as practicable from the vehicles. If you can do nothing else, drive to a telephone and ask the operator to put you in touch with the nearest police command.

2. If you're at the scene when the professionals arrive, get out of their way, offer to help and obey their instructions.

3. If you come upon an accident that already has emergency personnel at the scene, keep moving. Slow down so you have instant control of your car, but don't stop to gape. Mentally put yourself in the victim's place.

4. If you hear about an accident, on the radio for example, avoid the area. By the time you hear the news, the officials will already have taken charge and there'll be nothing you can do to help. Going there just for curiosity's sake will do more harm than good. And you may be among the losers.

Doctor Needed: When, Which, and How?

Alton L. Thygerson, Ed.D.

First aid means the emergency care given to an injured or ill person until medical care can be obtained. It is the obtaining of medical care which may pose one of the largest problems to the first-aider. For instance, the following questions will arise in all serious first aid cases: When do I call a doctor? Which doctor do I call? How do I call a doctor?

When to Call a Doctor?

People cannot run to a physician for every little bump, bruise, or hint of illness. If they did, doctors would be so occupied with minor complaints that they would have no time for major problems. It is necessary for adults to know the signs and symptoms of possible trouble and under what conditions their presence should send the victim to a physician.

Signs and symptoms are two different things: a sign is a visible evidence; a symptom is an internal feeling of the victim. Bleeding, vomiting, and a rapid pulse rate are signs because an observer (first-aider) can see or feel them. Headaches, earaches, fatigue, and nausea are symptoms because only the victim feels them. The first-aider knows of their existence through verbal questioning.

The American Medical Association (1) suggests four circumstances under which signs or symptoms demand prompt medical aid:

1. *Acuteness.* the signs or symptoms are too severe to be endured, i.e., sudden chest pains, abdominal pain, etc.

2. *Persistence.* a sign or a symptom persists for more than a few days or a week, i.e., itching, headaches, etc.

3. *Recurrence.* signs or symptoms return repeatedly without a clear-cut cause, i.e., digestive disturbances, etc.

4. *Unusualness.* whenever any sign or symptom raises doubts, it is safer to call the doctor than to take a chance.

Common signs which may be observed include bleeding, bowel changes, breathlessness, convulsions, cough, diarrhea, muscle spasms or cramps, paralysis, rashes, running ears, trembling, vomiting, and nonhealing sores.

Common symptoms include blackouts, constipation, dizziness, depression, earache, eyeache, fatigue, fever, headaches, itching, nausea, numbness, and pain.

It should be clear that using the above information is not diagnosing the problem. Signs and symptoms only identify a potential or possible problem which then needs to be diagnosed by a physician.

For instance in the obvious sign of bleeding there are times when a doctor should be called and other times when a doctor should *not* be called. Below are cases when a doctor should see a wound: (2)

1. There is spurting bleeding.
2. Slow bleeding continues beyond 4 to 10 minutes.
3. There is foreign material in the wound that does not wash out easily.
4. The wound is a deep puncture wound.
5. The wound is long or wide and thus may require stitches.
6. A nerve or tendon may be cut.
7. The wound is on the face or wherever else a noticeable scar would be undesirable.
8. The wound is of a type that cannot be completely cleansed.
9. The wound has been in contact with soil or manure.
10. The wound is an animal or human bite.
11. At the first sign of infection (pain, reddened area around wound, swelling).

Which Doctor to Call?

It should be obvious that for most emergency problems the family doctor should be called. The family doctor may be one of two choices: a general practitioner or a general internist. Both are trained medical doctors who can treat most emergencies.

There might be occasions arising when a specialist might be called. The specialist can be called in as a consultant by the family doctor or, if the victim has had similar, previous emergency problems involving a specialist, then a call directly to that specialist might be in order. An acute asthma attack, an emergency mental disturbance, or an emergency child birth situation are all times when a specialist — here an allergist, psychiatrist, or obstetrician — might be utilized.

If you are vacationing or have moved away from your family doctor when an emergency arises, you have two choices. One is to go to what appears to be the best general hospital available. For example, there are usually freeway road signs marking exits to the nearest hospital. The other choice is to phone the local medical society, tell them your problem and ask them to suggest a physician. Some hotels and motels can offer suggestions about doctors or may even have a resident physician. In some 500 communities in the United States, another answer is the Doctor's Emergency Service (DES) (3). The telephone number for the DES is found either on the inside front cover of a phone directory or it may be found in the Yellow Pages under "Physicians and Surgeons (M.D.)."

How to Call a Doctor?

It may seem very elementary to talk about how to call a doctor. It is taught to children at the elementary school level and should be taught by parents to their children for the unexpected emergency. It is simple; you pick up the telephone and call him.

Nevertheless, take the case of a worried relative who calls the doctor and is so excited that she screams into the phone to come quick, Sam is dying, and then hangs up before giving the necessary information. In other cases the doctor is called but is given no information as to what to expect when he gets there.

When a physician is called, the *who*, the *where*, and the *what* are important:

1. *Who?* Is the victim a child or an elderly person. Also the caller's name and telephone number should be given for possible questions which may arise in the physician's mind or in case of difficulty in locating the address given by the caller.

2. *Where?* Is it nearby or in a remote area. Possibly the first-aider transporting the victim to a hospital would be quicker and more expedient than having a doctor attempt to locate an unfamiliar address or location.

3. *What?* Give the signs and symptoms of the problem.

If you have not had the experience of calling a doctor in an emergency situation, you will have in the future. With one in four Americans accidentally injured yearly, along with the other illnesses arising, it is best to be prepared in advance for calling your doctor. Have his telephone number or numbers and those of an alternate doctor in an accessible place.

A decision must be made by the first-aider regarding how the medical care can best be obtained. Consultation with a physician on a telephone will most often determine how the victim can best obtain medical aid. A choice is usually from among the following:

1. *Transport.* Transporting the victim to the doctor or the hospital is commonly done, wisely or sometimes unwisely, depending upon the injury and illness, by using the automobile. It might depend upon the automobile's condition, distance to medical aid, and number of responsible assistants. For many injuries and illnesses the ambulance is the answer (i.e., spinal cord injuries). The ambulance may also best handle those problems dealing with the factors mentioned above such as assistants, etc. Success with ambulance helicopters in Vietnam and Korea has led to their introduction for handling medical emergencies in many metropolitan and remote areas.

2. *Summon.* Because of the severity of a broken bone or other injuries and illnesses, the doctor may be summoned to the home or injury scene. This is usually best determined by the doctor after the first-aider has communicated to him the signs, symptoms, and other information which may be pertinent to the individual case.

3. *Wait.* In some cases the injury or illness may not require immediate medical care. Thus, the first-aider can receive telephoned information from the doctor about caring for the victim to see if improvement and progress toward better health is achieved, or to bide time until a doctor or an emergency vehicle

arrives, which in some locales takes considerable time (i.e., wilderness areas and remote stretches of highways).

It should be clear that the telephone is usually accessible for obtaining information from a physician and for summoning an ambulance or a doctor. However, there are times when the lack of a telephone may necessitate the sending of a responsible person for assistance or even the commandeering of a vehicle for transportation. Another communication method of seeking assistance is through the use of distress signals such as SOS, three gunshots, or three smoke fires.

The phase of first aid contained in this article is often complicated by emotional pressure, inexperience, and the pressure of time. Therefore, take the necessary time and effort to obtain immediate medical aid by a physician. Further injury can develop during the interval of time between the initiation of first aid procedures and the arrival of medical care, for which the first-aider can be responsible and thus negligent.

REFERENCES

1. Amercan Medical Association. "When To Call Your Doctor." *Today's Health*, October 1966.
2. American Medical Association. "Emergency First Aid." *Today's Health Guide*. Chicago: The Association, 1965, p. 349.
3. Irwin, Theodore. "I Need a Doctor." *Today's Health*, October 1968, pp. 35-37.

Legal Considerations in First Aid

Alton L. Thygerson, Ed.D.

Approximately one in every four Americans suffers an accident of some degree each year (1). Thus, the chances for a person to confront an injured victim are quite real and even probable in view of the above-stated statistic.

Seldom mentioned or discussed in first aid texts are the problems of negligence and its legal ramifications, which are centered upon a question often asked in first aid classes and in the minds of all who may administer emergency care — Can I be sued if I render first aid? The main purpose of this treatise is not to develop lawyers but to guide the first-aider in some legal phases of first aid. Hopefully, the important question "Can I be sued if I render first aid?" will be answered so that first-aiders will continue to provide the needed and valuable service of rendering aid to the injured and sick.

Negligence is complex and often confusing. Therefore, in most cases, a judge and jury would make the final decision in each particular case. In essence, negligence is the *failure to act as a reasonably prudent person would act under the particular circumstances*. Factors in the definition lead to these concepts:

1. *Failure to Act.* Negligence can consist of acts of commission or omission. If one fails to do something expected of him by law, he can be negligent. The law expects first aid to be rendered to injured students by teachers (2), to the public by police, to traffic accident victims by those involved, although it should be pointed out that there is no law requiring one person to assist a stranger. For example, a good swimmer may stand and watch another person drown a short distance away. A physician is not required to help nonpatients who may be dying and who might be saved by him. However, both the good swimmer and the physician who fail to help another human being will have the rest of their lives to reflect upon a decision which may prove difficult to live with. Remember, as stated before, certain occupations require first aid training and the administering of proper first aid to those injured.

2. *A Reasonably Prudent Person.* A volunteer first-aider offering assistance to an injured person must use reasonable care. Certainly a victim may sue a first-aider, but such suits are nearly nonexistent and are almost always thrown out of court. It is hard to believe that the courts would go so far as to permit an injured person to collect liability damages from one who tried to assist or render first aid, unless there were evidence of willful carelessness or misconduct while handling the injured person.

The standards for a reasonably prudent first-aider are in the procedures found in Red Cross manuals, Boy Scout handbooks, etc. If a first-aider invents his own procedures and techniques for treating a first aid problem, then negligence might be found. To illustrate, two teachers held a student's infected hand in scalding water, causing blisters and permanent disfigurement. Both were deemed negligent (3).

The following may serve as general guidelines and summary for the first-aider:

1. A person is under no legal obligation to assist an injured person whom he meets. The exceptions are in certain occupations where it is part of one's job to render first aid and in traffic accident situations.

2. When a first-aider gives help, he must do so with reasonable skill in order to avoid further injury to the already existing injury. For instance, if a simple fracture becomes compounded through carelessness or willful misconduct, negligence exists.

3. A person can volunteer first aid, but no one can order or compel a first-aider to render aid.

4. The first-aider should remain with the victim after starting emergency care until the injured is turned over to a qualified doctor, another first-aider (i.e., ambulance technician, etc.), or a relative.

5. The first-aider should use standard first-aid methods — not invented procedures or techniques.

6. A person should never force treatment on anyone except in three hurried cases: severe bleeding, absence of breathing, and poisoning.

A lesser problem in first-aid situations is the liability of medical personnel (physicians and nurses) for rendering first aid in emergency situations. A literature search has found no case in which a doctor or nurse has been held liable for giving first aid to an accident victim at the accident scene.

To protect physicians from malpractice suits due to rendering first aid, "good samaritan" laws were adopted in many states. Such laws do not seem to give physicians and nurses any greater protection than that already existing under common law. If doctors and nurses were more familiar with the already existing protection, the need for "good samaritan" laws would disappear (4).

REFERENCES

1. "Accidental Death and Disability: The Neglected Disease of Modern Society." National Academy of Sciences, 1966, p. 6.
2. Trubitt, Hillard J. "Legal Responsibilities of School Teachers in Emergency Situations." *Journal of School Health*, January 1966, p. 26.
3. Guerrieri v. Tyson, 24 A. (2d) 468 (Pennsylvania, 1942).
4. Henderson, Gordon F., and Fisk, George. "To Help or Not To Help — a Nurse's Dilemma." *The Canadian Nurse*, February 1968.

Psychological First Aid

Darwin K. Gillespie, Ph.D.

In 1947, two freighters loaded with nitrates blew up and flattened Texas City. 570 people were killed. Every building within one-half mile of the blast was destroyed. Chunks of hot metal weighing several thousand pounds were thrown like mortar shells some two miles. The streets were crowded with panicky people. One witness reported that a kind of "shellshock" madness seized the town. About 3,000 people were given psychological first aid by Red Cross, military, and other people. There weren't enough medics to go around nor was there time for elaborate treatment. First aid was the order of the day.

In a classroom at "X" school, a pupil was accused of cheating on an examination. When confronted with the evidence the pupil "went to pieces" and began to cry hysterically. The teacher handed a candy mint to the pupil and said in a calm voice, "Why was this test so important to you?" A little self-control became apparent in the pupil.

One out of every five casualties in the Korean conflict was psychological. Nearly 80% of these were restored to constructive effort by psychological first aid administered in the combat zone. At the same rate of casualty production, if a hydrogen bomb were dropped on a major city such as New York City, one could expect more than a million emotional casualties among those who were far enough away from ground zero to escape physical harm. Fear, apprehension, and anxiety may likely spread to other cities in a sort of chain reaction.

These instances point out the need for developing in the general population some understanding of the fundamental principles of dealing with psychologically disturbed or disorganized persons. Medical help at times of severe community disaster must be augmented by individuals from the general population who can intelligently administer first aid not only to those with physical injuries but to those suffering from emotional trauma.

There are several places in our health curriculum that could offer information on how to deal effectively with depressed, overactive, terrified disaster victims who are not physically injured. One of these is the "First Aid" course and another is the unit on "Disaster and Civil Defense." Applicability of the principles to individual situations in the family or school or elsewhere should suggest other areas within the health curriculum. Logically, the mental health units could contain this kind of information in support of one's emotional resistance in meeting the stress of a difficult situation. Knowing what to expect and what to do is a sound antidote for anxiety.

Reprinted with permission from *American Journal of School Health*, November 1963, Vol. 33, No. 9, pp. 391-395.

Psychological first aid can be briefly and effectively presented by first considering the kinds of reactions to be expected from a situation producing gross stress, and second what should the first-aider do or not do in these instances. The chart is presented to show a convenient way to organize these ideas.

Reaction to sudden disaster may be classified into five types:
1. Normal conduct
2. Panic
3. Depression
4. Over-activity
5. Physical reactions

Even under very severe conditions some people can remain calm, poised, and effective. Most of us, however, will reveal some signs of anxiety. We may shake, feel weak, be nauseated, and perspire excessively. We may not be able to think clearly. These reactions are transient and usually we can regain some control of ourselves. It is apparent that such people need very little first aid. A little reassurance such as an encouraging comment or a pat on the shoulder will generally help the return of self-control. A good general rule is that psychological first aid is necessary only for those people who have lost, or are losing, their self-control and are making no noticeable progress toward regaining normal functions.

The chief characteristic of panic is blind flight. Judgment seems to disappear in panicky people and in their frantic effort to get away they may physically harm themselves. When such frantic attempts to run away occur in groups of highly emotional people the reaction becomes dangerous because it is contagious and can easily stampede others who ordinarily would stand fast but who are temporarily disorganized. Panic reaction may also be evident in those who cry uncontrollably or pointlessly demonstrate wild physical activity. (Standard textbooks in social psychology present such phenomena under the title of "crowd behavior" or "mob psychology.") The panic reaction is least responsive to psychological first aid. It is often difficult to get the attention of these people. In order to avoid group panic, it is very important to segregate and control these individuals. Get help from others in taking this kind of a reactant to some medical facility. Don't try to do it yourself because if he breaks away from you he will be even more disturbed. If you can't get him to a medical facility, assign some people to stay with him. Physical restraint may be necessary. Such restraint should be firm — not brutal or punitive. Do not slap a person in panic, nor should you douse him with cold water. Harsh and abusive measures may halt disorganized behavior temporarily but it will intensify his anxiety of those nearby who may be on the verge of panic themselves.

In the depressed reaction, the individual draws back into himself as a protection against more stress. Some will act as though they were numbed. They may sit or stand in the middle of destruction as if completely oblivious to the impact

PSYCHOLOGICAL FIRST AID FOR DISASTER REACTIONS

Reactions	Symptoms	Do	Don't

Normal	Trembling
	Muscular tension
	Perspiration
	Nausea
	Mild diarrhea
	Urinary frequency
	Pounding heart
	Rapid breathing
	Anxiety
		Give reassurance
		Provide group
		  identification
		Motivate
		Talk with him
		Observe to see that
		  individual is
		  gaining composure
		  not losing it
			Don't show
			  resentment
			Don't overdo
			  sympathy

Individual
  Panic
  (flight-
  reaction)
	Unreasoning attempt
	  to flee
	Loss of judgment
	Uncontrolled
	  weeping
	Wild running about
		Try kindly firmness
		  at first
		Give something
		  warm to eat or
		  drink
		Get help to isolate,
		  if necessary
		Be empathetic
		Encourage him to
		  talk
		Be aware of your
		  own limitations
			Don't use brutal
			  restraint
			Don't strike
			Don't douse with
			  water
			Don't give
			  sedatives

Depression
  (Underactive
  reactions)
	Stand or sit without
	  moving or talking
	Vacant expression
	Lack of emotional
	  display
		Get contact gently
		Secure rapport
		Get them to tell you
		  what happened
		Be empathetic
		Recognize feelings
		  of resentment in
		  patient and your-
		  self
		Find simple, routine
		  job
		Give warm food,
		  drink
			Don't tell them to
			  "snap out of it"
			Don't overdo pity
			Don't give
			  sedatives
			Don't act
			  resentful

Overactive	Argumentative
	Talk rapidly
	Joke inappropriately
	Make endless
	  suggestions
	Jump from one
	  activity to another
		Let them talk about
		  it
		Find them jobs
		  which require
		  physical effort
		Give warm food,
		  drink
		Supervision necessary
		Be aware of own
		  feelings
			Don't suggest that
			  they are acting
			  abnormally
			Don't give
			  sedatives
			Don't argue with
			  them

PSYCHOLOGICAL FIRST AID FOR DISASTER REACTIONS

Reactions	Symptoms	Do	Don't
Physical (Conversion reaction)	Severe nausea and vomiting Can't use some part of the body	Show interest in them Find small job for them to make them forget Make comfortable Get medical help if possible Be aware of own feelings	Don't tell them that there's nothing wrong with them Don't blame Don't ridicule Ignore disability openly

Modified from M 51-400-603-1, Dept. of Non-resident Instruction, Medical Field Service School, Brooke Army Medical Center, Fort Sam Houston, Texas.

of the situation. When spoken to they may not reply. They cannot help themselves. The best first aid for this type is calm and realistic assurance. A few moments spent with each individual or with several in a small group will bring desirable results in many of them. A few moments of understanding will pave the way for positive suggestion or a simple suggestion to do a specific task. If children are in the area they are likely to respond to the attitudes of adults around them.

In contrast to the depressed, some individuals will be overly active. Their great show of activity may at first glance appear to be purposeful, but upon closer observation it will appear to be quite senseless. Rapid speech is characteristic. Sometimes these people will offer suggestions which are of little value and inappropriate. They may be unrealistically self-confident and be unable to take direction from others. This type of response can breed danger because the person may be able to gather support from others in opposing sound procedures which must be put into effect. Although it may be difficult, at first, to get through to them, these people will pay some attention to you. The first-aider should guide them into doing useful work such as walking another person to a shelter, digging out casualties, moving debris, directing traffic, etc. Do not argue with these people. They are prone to criticize.

Physical reactions to stress may be so severe as to involve loss of sight, hearing, speech, use of a limb, or total immobility without physical cause. Such a condition is technically known as conversion reaction. Thus, a person unconsciously converts his anxiety into a strong belief that some part, or all, of his body has ceased to function. These people are just as disabled as if they had a physical injury. They are aware that there is no physical basis for their symptoms but they are unable to correct the situation themselves. The first-aider should speak calmly and reassuringly to these individuals. Make them feel that you are interested in them. Try to find some small job for them which can be performed in spite of their symptoms. This will give them a chance to regain their composure gradually while waiting for medical assistance.

Although the basic principles of psychological first aid are not always easy to apply, a great amount of good can be done by following these simple guidelines:

1. Recognize emotional injury in a person.
2. Obtain rapport. Get through to the casualty. Get him to understand that you want to help. This may be the toughest part of the job. An emotional casualty is often so saturated with fear that he trusts no one, not even his friends. He sees danger in everything and puts up a wall to protect himself. The job of the first-aider is to break down this wall. The casualty needs to know that he isn't alone and that you want to help him. He needs understanding, however, more than sympathy.
3. Let him talk out his feelings and fears. This is the biggest bit of help you can offer. Little by little he talks away the fear and his world begins to take shape again.
4. Sleep is an excellent first aid tool. When a person is exhausted, sleep can work miracles. It seems to bring back strength and self-control almost over night. When the casualty awakens give him something to do. This will tend to get his mind off the stresses which pushed him under. Make him feel that he is worthwhile and that he is needed.
5. Sometimes the procedures in the fourth step have to be reversed. An emotionally wound up person may not be settled enough to sleep for some time in spite of calm reassurances. A few hours of work or other physical activity can calm him and give him an outlet for his agitation so that sleep can come naturally.

It is important to remember that sedatives should not be administered to a psychological casualty unless given under the direction of a physician or other qualified person. Emotionally bound people are muddled in their thinking and a sedative may only add to their confusion. Furthermore, a sedative may make the casualty inaccessible to first aid treatment.

Summary

As many people as possible should gain an understanding of psychological first aid. A general understanding can reduce the emotional effects of a community disaster and it can serve the individual as a strong emotional support in a crisis. The school health curriculum provides excellent opportunities for developing many individuals capable of providing appropriate first aid care for those with emotional wounds. The procedures are easy to remember; obtain rapport, get him to talk, give him something to do, and allow him to sleep if he needs it.

REFERENCES

1. Office of Civil and Defense Mobilization. *Disaster Readiness in Undergraduate Education*. Battle Creek, Michigan, 1960.
2. LaPiere, R.T., and P.R. Farnsworth. *Social Psychology*. 3rd ed. New York: McGraw-Hill Book Company, 1949, Ch. 25.
3. Meerloo, A.M. *Patterns of Panic*. New York: International University Press, 1950.

Why Must Crash Victims Die?

James R. Miller

A young soldier steps on a land mine in Vietnam and a young civilian steps in front of a speeding car in a large Midwestern city. Both of them suffer grave multiple injuries. Only one of them has an excellent chance of survival.

Which one?

The solider — no doubt about it.

This is not recruiting propaganda. It is sober medical opinion. Although the fourth greatest killer in this country is accidental physical injury, few U.S. hospitals can cope with it as expertly as a medical unit in a combat area.

Recently some 300 physicians and other interested persons met in Washington to discuss this kind of injury and how to handle it. Their word for it — "trauma" — covers all of the states of disrepair caused by blows, cuts, blasts, falls, shocks, poisons and burns. But what they focused on can be described simply as physical injury, usually accidental, that is severe enough to put the victim out of action and present a threat to his life.

The size of the problem was underscored by their reference to trauma as being "epidemic" and "the nation's most important environmental health problem." These were not overstatements. Consider:

• Annually in the U.S. alone, about 50 million accidental injuries account for 115,000 dead, 400,000 permanently impaired, and 10.5 million temporarily disabled. Accident victims occupy 65,000 hospital beds for 22 million bed-days.

• Only heart disease, cancer and stroke cause more deaths, and even these are outranked by accident in the 1 to 37 age group. Accidents cause well over 40 percent of all deaths of children between the ages of 1 and 15.

• Nearly half of the accidental deaths involve motor vehicles. About a quarter of them occur in the home, and an eighth at work.

• The annual cost to Americans — quite apart from the immeasurable anguish — totals $25 billion. This includes medical expenses, wage losses, insurance costs and property damage. It is roughly equal to annual appropriation for the war in Vietnam.

One of the more frustrating aspects of the accidental injury problem is that of prevention. Accidents are commonly the result of our own clumsiness, carelessness and cussedness. And there is much more that can be done about it in the safer design of vehicles, factory equipment and household appliances, in the engineering of roads and the inspection of cars, in the scrutiny and testing of

Reprinted with permission from *Family Safety*, Vol. 29, No. 4, Winter 1970, pp. 12-15. Copyright © 1970 by The Reader's Digest Association, Inc.

new drugs, in general education of the public. But this is a long-range goal, and for this reason the doctors in Washington concentrated on how best to deal with the injury once it has occurred.

We may wonder why in a country boasting the best medical people and facilities in the world, the handling of accident victims leaves so much to be desired. One of the main reasons, as stressed in a 1966 report by the Division of Medical Sciences of the National Academy of Sciences/National Research Council, is the gap between knowledge and application. Talent and good will abound, but often the efforts of even the ablest people are not properly orchestrated for the job at hand.

For a man who falls off his roof or tangles with a power saw four elements of assistance are needed immediately: first aid, fast transportation, effective communications, a good emergency medical facility.

Offhand, it might seem that all four could reasonably be taken for granted. In most American communities not even one of these elements can be. The average citizen has had little, if any, first-aid training. And yet the first aid required in this kind of predicament is advanced first aid, reflecting the knowledge of what to do and what not to do about fractures, hemorrhage and impaired breathing. With serious injury, the first 15 to 30 minutes are critical.

The best hope, then, is that an ambulance will arrive soon with one or more skilled attendants who can give the patient expert attention on the spot and on the way to a medical center. Unhappily, you can't take this for granted either. To quote the report of the Division of Medical Sciences: "First-class ambulance service exists in few cities. There are no generally accepted standards for the competence and training of ambulance attendants. Attendants may be unschooled apprentices lacking training in even elementary first aid." Untold thousands die or are permanently disabled by inadequately trained ambulance and rescue crews.

As for the ambulances themselves: "Approximately 50 percent of the country's ambulance services are provided by 12,000 morticians, mainly because their vehicles can accommodate litters. No manufacturer produces from the assembly line a vehicle that can be termed an ambulance (with low floor and high dome, for example, so the attendants can work on their feet). Most ambulances in this country are impractical for resuscitative care, have incomplete fixed equipment, and carry inadequate supplies."

There is no lack of information on how to improve this picture. The U.S. Public Health Service offers comprehensive manuals on the requirements for ambulance design and equipment and on the training of ambulance personnel.

Now let's consider the third element in emergency management — communications.

The Division of Medical Sciences reports laconically: "Although it is possible to converse with astronauts in outer space, communication is seldom possible between an ambulance and the emergency department it is approaching."

It is hard to imagine anything more obvious than this need. The ambulance attendant should be able to alert the hospital for an admission, to report on the victim's condition, tell what he's doing for him and receive advice. He should also be able to reach the police and fire departments who can clear traffic lanes for him and mobilize additional rescue equipment.

But, with rare exceptions, ambulance radios (if any) provide communication only between the driver and his dispatcher, and hospitals are usually notified of an accident by local radio or television, or by a phone call from the police or the walking wounded.

As for the emergency facility, assuming a man has been injured, that he has received some kind of first aid and that he is now in an ambulance and on his way, we can ask, on his way to what?

More than likely to the "nearest" hospital. In many communities, it is the set policy of ambulance operators to go to the nearest hospital regardless of whether it is the one best able to handle the case.

Ninety percent of the 7000 accredited hospitals in the United States provide "emergency rooms." In general, they are small and poorly equipped. They are understaffed, usually having on hand one attendant and one intern. Many of these emergency rooms cannot even pretend to the capability their name implies and are often little more than outpatient clinics crowded by people with head colds and sprained ankles. Of the 40 million emergency room visits in 1966, fewer than one third were truly emergencies. To make matters worse, these rooms are shortest of staff on nights and holidays and weekends when a great percentage of serious accidents occur.

Clearly much could be done to improve the lot of the accident victim. The requirements for ambulance services are tough but not beyond the resources of most communities. They can best be met, doctors argue, if our communities look upon the ambulances as a "third service," alongside the police and fire departments, to be supported, as the other two are, by community taxes. The equipment should be every bit as good as that used by policemen and firemen. The ambulance attendants should have equally intensive training, comparable wage scales and security provisions. Also recommended is a much wider use of helicopter ambulances, especially for service in rural areas and towns of 2500 and under, where nearly 70 percent of our traffic fatalities occur. Helicopters in Vietnam take an average of only 17 minutes to move a wounded man from where he is struck down to a forward aid station. Two helicopters operated by the Arizona Department of Public Safety last year flew 225 patients from all over the state to regional emergency facilities.

Finally, the doctors are now endorsing an ambitious scheme to upgrade the

emergency medical centers themselves. The essence of it is categorization –
reducing emergency facilities in some hospitals, increasing them in others, to
provide an integrated network with four categories:

1. Advanced First-Aid Facility. Part-time physician and nursing staff.
Capable of handling minor injuries. (Most existing hospital emergency rooms are
in this category.)

2. Limited Emergency Facility. A nurse and perhaps a physician always
available, but no ready access to specialists. Adequate in many cases, but could
best serve critically injured by emphasis on resuscitation and preparation for
transfer to center with greater resources.

3. Major Emergency Facility. Physicians and nurses, highly trained in lifesaving methods, available 24 hours a day. Specialists always on call. Must have
blood bank, complete resuscitative equipment, X-ray instruments, around-the-
clock laboratory services and immediate access to operating rooms. Should be
integral element of a large hospital and university medical center.

4. Emergency Facility and Trauma Research Unit. This is the ideal, combin-
ing everything in the third category with an intensive program of research in
support of therapy.

All of this is a big order, and no one can even look at it without wondering
about the price tag. Efficiency in the treatment of trauma victims will cost
heavily, the doctors admit. But they insist that the cost should be borne – not
only for humanitarian reasons but because the long-run economic saving would
be immense.

One might also wonder whether, given the money, medical people are really
able to create the kind of emergency service they envision, whether they can
close the gap between knowledge and application.

You can bet that they can.

One day recently, at 2:10 p.m., a 22-year-old man lost control of his car on
a highway curve and rolled it off the shoulder at 60 m.p.h.

His injuries were appalling, but this accident happened in Baltimore, Md., a
city that is superbly prepared for this kind of casualty.

A cruising state trooper saw the car and called the Valley Post of the state
police, which in turn summoned to the site one of their two helicopters, and also
on their direct line, called the Center for the Study of Trauma at the University
of Maryland Hospital in downtown Baltimore. Several other hospitals were
nearer, but Baltimore, unlike most communities, was geared to get him to the
best. At 2:17 the helicopter landed the patient on the roof of a building adjoining the hospital. He was rolled down a ramp and into the trauma center. Time of
arrival: 2:25 p.m.

The room he entered has no superior in this country when it comes to
emergency treatment. It is a square room, 50 by 50 feet, dominated by a raised
center island from which doctors and nurses can keep their eyes on each of the

12 patient cubicles that surround it. It is manned continuously (24 hours a day, 365 days a year) by two or more physicians and five or six nurses. Every patient area contains an armamentarium of lifesaving equipment: respirators, catheters, probes and sensors for blood vessels and vital organs, data-monitoring systems that can signal micropumps to force needed fluids or medications fast. Each area's monitoring scopes for pulse rate, blood pressure and heart output are duplicated on the center island.

Today's patient needed all the help he could get. On admission he was scarcely breathing, his blood pressure was dangerously low and he was in a deep coma. The onset of shock appeared imminent, and Dr. Paul Hanashiro, clinical director of the trauma unit, mounted a maximum effort to head it off, ordering intravenous injection of salt solution to replace lost fluids and the placement of a tube in the trachea to establish an airway. X-rays revealed fractures of three ribs, the left shoulder blade, plus a broken back. Orthopedists and neurosurgeons were called in at once.

The patient remained unconscious for four days. Given the ordinary circumstances — slow transportation to a run-of-the-mill hospital — he would surely have died. He is now on the way to recovery.

In fact, of more than 300 gravely injured patients hurried to this trauma center in the past 12 months, 225 recovered. With ordinary treatment, doctors believe that at least half of the survivors would have died.

Although the Center for the Study of Trauma has only 12 beds, most of them normally occupied, it is still one of the largest emergency facilities in the world, and it took a lot of doing to bring it into existence. In 1966, the National Institute of General Medical Sciences (a division of the National Institutes of Health) became so concerned about trauma that it decided to offer grants for research to several hospitals that showed particular promise of carrying it out successfully. There are now eight Trauma Research Centers. One of them is the University of Maryland Hospital (affiliated with the University of Maryland School of Medicine) where, since 1961, a pilot clinical shock unit had been operating under the direction of Dr. R. Adams Cowley, now chief of thoracic and cardiovascular surgery at the hospital. Starting with the concept of a 12-bed patient area, Dr. Cowley and his colleagues designed the five-story, $2-million unit that opened its doors for services in June, 1969. Here Dr. Cowley now supervises a multidisciplinary team of about 70 surgeons, internists, biochemists, bacteriologists, computer specialists, bioelectronics engineers and nurses. The Baltimore organization clearly represents dramatic progress in trauma therapy and research. Today doctors from other institutions are being rotated on its staff, and last year more than 100 came to observe and study the center's operation.

Obviously, not all communities can afford such a facility. But many more can than do. Money is essential. So are will and leadership on all sides — on the part of doctors for clear reasons; on the part of industry, which loses hundreds of millions of dollars each year because of disabled employes; on the part of insurance companies, which pay the claims; and finally, on the part of the taxpayers themselves. After all, none of us leads a charmed life.

First Aid for Cardiopulmonary Emergencies

Mouth-to-Mouth Resuscitation—
Isn't It Worth the Risk?

Ronald L. Linder

Mouth-to-mouth artificial respiration, practiced from biblical days up until it fell prey to Pasteur's germ theory during the late 1800's A.D., is again under consideration. (1) The risk of acquiring infectious disease in mouth-to-mouth breathing is a target of recent concern. Let us examine the facts before discarding the newly reinstituted mouth-to-mouth method of resuscitation.

A case of primary cutaneous tuberculosis resulting from oral resuscitation is reported in one of the latest issues of *The New England Journal of Medicine.* (5) A 25-year-old intern in the Second (Cornell) Medical Division at Bellevue Hospital contracted primary cutaneous tuberculosis (near the mouth) following mouth-to-mouth resuscitation of a patient who stopped breathing shortly after admission. Postmortem examination of the patient disclosed active tuberculosis of the right upper lobe. Approximately eight weeks after his contact the intern noted a slightly tender area, which later developed into a lesion on the left side of his face near the nose. A biopsy revealed tubercle bacilli. No preventive measures were taken by the intern prior to the biopsy.

This case certainly confirms the necessity for the operator to seek medical guidance following resuscitation. The cooperation of physicians and hospital personnel in providing the operator with pertinent information and guidance is essential. In mouth-to-mouth resuscitation, the fear of cross-infection and other objections based on hygienic, psychological, social, sexual or racial grounds are difficult for some individuals to ignore. However, not until the last decade has such an abundance of research data supported the superiority of the oral resuscitation method and demonstrated the ineffectiveness of all previously practiced manual methods. (1)

In an experiment involving ten anesthetized and curarized adult volunteers and ten apneic patients mouth-to-mouth resuscitation was effective in moving volumes of air greater than 1500 ml., while the Silvestor (prone-pressure) and the Holger-Nielsen (back-pressure-arm-lift) manual methods were effective only in moving deadspace air in 50% of the trials. (8)

In studies conducted by Gordon and others (4) using the manual back-pressure-arm-lift method and the manual rocking method, total blockage of the air passage was observed in all of the remaining subjects.

Dill (2) states, "Obstruction of the airway above the larynx is the most common cause of failure of any method of artificial respiration. In expired-air

Reprinted with permission from *American Journal of School Health*, April 1967, Vol. 37, No. 4, pp. 187-189.

breathing, this type of obstruction is prevented, for the hands are free to keep the head extended at the atlantoccipital (sniffing position) and the lower jaw displaced forward."

All methods of artificial respiration have certain disadvantages; however, the advantages of mouth-to-mouth resuscitation far exceed its disadvantages for the following reasons (7, 2, 4, 8, 1):

1. The mouth-to-mouth method is superior to all manual methods in assuring the major function of resuscitation — pulmonary ventilation.
2. Since air passage obstruction is the most common cause of inadequate ventilation the supremacy of mouth-to-mouth resuscitation, enabling the operator constantly to monitor the air passage to insure ventilation, cannot be overemphasized.
3. Mouth-to-mouth resuscitation requires less energy expenditure even when the victim is much larger than the rescuer.
4. Mouth-to-mouth resuscitation is a universal method which can be performed by and on all ages and sizes.
5. Equipment or adjuncts are not essential to the proper performance of mouth-to-mouth resuscitation.
6. If closed heart massage is necessary the mouth-to-mouth technique of resuscitation best facilitates this procedure. Since adequate pulmonary ventilation without serious circulatory impairment is the most important criterion of the resuscitative technique to be used, mouth-to-mouth resuscitation is the most effective procedure, as it "assures adequate ventilation in all cases."
7. Research has conclusively supported the superiority of the mouth-to-mouth method in maintaining adequate oxygenation and carbon dioxide elimination for prolonged periods.

Elam and others (3) report, "Extensive physiological measurements in 29 adult anesthetized patients demonstrate expired air resuscitation to be an efficient, versatile method of artificial respiration. Reoxygenation of the patient's lungs is possible with four inflations, and within a circulation time arterial oxygen saturation can be restored to normal. Carbon dioxide levels are concomitantly reduced."

Current findings support the belief that in most cases irreversible central nervous system damage begins within four or five minutes after submersion in victims who suffer heart stoppage. Since the rescuer is unable to determine when the "threshold of death" is reached (estimates vary from 5 to 10 minutes), it is imperative that he should begin mouth-to-mouth resuscitation on the unconscious victim in the water. A delay may result only in recovering a corpse. (6)

"The teachability of mouth-to-mouth breathing is demonstrated by the fact that 90% of 164 untrained rescuers performed this method satisfactorily after one demonstration. Women and children who weigh 45.4 kg. (100 lb.) can ventilate adequately victims who weigh approximately 91 kg. (200 lb.)." (7)

Several investigators have recommended the use of suitable adjuncts to oral resuscitation in an effort to surmount the various objections to the mouth-to-mouth method. Safar (8) indicates several advantages of the *mouth-to-airway* technique over the direct mouth-to-mouth technique:

1. Better pulmonary ventilation
2. More acceptable to the operator
3. Less gastric distention of the victim
4. Less fatiguing to the rescuer
5. Fewer failures, because maintenance of a patent upper airway is easier

Brooks and others (1) also support the mouth-to-airway technique since a suitable airway improves airway patency and provides an effective seal against leakage, which is a problem when the operator's lips are applied to the victim's mouth which is kept open to allow the exchange of air.

A fundamental question follows — which airway device is suitable? The answer is as varied as the vast number of different airway devices available. The lack of unanimity with respect to a suitable airway device which is portable, simple, inexpensive, easily applied, safe for the victim and protective for the operator is evidenced throughout the medical literature. Suppose an airway device were developed that had been given the stamp of approval by most physicians. How many persons could and would carry such an airway at all times? The answer appears obvious — very few. How many persons you know keep an airway device in their "pocket, glove compartment or bag, ready to help save lives in emergencies?"

Since the majority of stoppage-of-breathing catastrophes occur outside the hospital and the physician's office, and since the victim's life often depends on prompt effective resuscitation by the first person to arrive at the scene of the emergency, the practicality of using the airway technique exclusively is questionable. However, the training of personnel of rescue units, first aid rooms, and swimming areas for example in the mouth-to-airway technique would be advisable.

It is interesting to note that few investigators have raised the question of the victim acquiring an infectious disease from the operator. At this point a familiar statement used often in teaching first aid care for severe bleeding bears repeating: "It is better to have a live man with dirty wounds than a dead man with clean wounds." Nevertheless the direction of transmission of disease is or ought to be immaterial.

We are now left with the problem of what to do on those occasions of need when one discovers he has forgotten his airway at home. Since the victim usually has no choice in the method of resuscitation used, the decision rests completely with the first-aider. An inescapable values question is all that remains. Is the chance a person takes of acquiring an infectious disease (which in most cases would be curable) when administering oral resuscitation worth the possibility of saving the life of a fellow man?

REFERENCES

1. Brook, Joseph, Brook, M.H., and Lopez, J.F. "Artificial Respiration and Artificial Circulation." *The Canadian Medical Association Journal,* 1965, pp. 93, 396.
2. Dill, D.M. "Council on Medical Physics, Symposium on Mouth-to-Mouth Resuscitation (Expired Air Inflation)." *Journal of The American Medical Association,* 1958, pp. 167, 317.
3. Elam, J.O., Greene, D.G., Brown, E.S., and Clements, J.A. "Council on Medical Physics, Symposium on Mouth-to-Mouth Resuscitation (Expired Air Inflation) Oxygen and Carbon Dioxide Exchange and Energy Cost of Expired Air Resuscitation." *Journal of The American Medical Association,* 1958, pp. 167, 328.
4. Gordon, A.S., Frye, C.W., Bittelson, L., Sadove, M.S., and Beattie, E.J., Jr. "Council on Medical Physics, Symposium on Mouth-to-Mouth Resuscitation (Expired Air Inflation), Mouth-to-Mouth Versus Manual Artificial Respiration for Children and Adults." *Journal of The American Medical Association,* 1958, pp. 167, 320.
5. Heilman, K.M., and Muchenheim, C. "Primary Cutaneous Tuberculosis Resulting from Mouth-to-Mouth Respiration: Report of a Case." *The New England Journal of Medicine,* 1966, 273, pp. 1035-36.
6. Imburg, J., and Hartney, T. "Drowning and the Treatment of Non-fatal Submersion." *Pediatrics,* 1966, 37, pp. 684-698.
7. Safar, P. "Council on Medical Physics, Symposium on Mouth-to-Mouth Resuscitation (Expired Air Inflation), Ventilatory Efficacy of Mouth-to-Mouth Artificial Respiration." *Journal of The American Medical Association,* 1958, pp. 167, 335.
8. _____. "Mouth-to-Mouth Airway." *Anesthesiology,* 1957, pp. 18, 906.

The Tragedy of Needless Drowning Deaths

George Upton

Each year, more than 6000 people lose their lives in fresh and salt water drownings. Many of these drownings occur at supervised beaches and pools where the personnel on duty attempt rescue procedures which prove to be insufficient. It is generally thought that these victims are beyond the point of a successful rescue, and no questions are asked about the rescue procedures used, or whether additional steps could have been taken to revive the victims.

Within the past few years various research articles have appeared in the *Journal of the American Medical Association (JAMA)*, dealing with the physiology of drowning and the rescue procedures that should be used on the drowning victim. These articles indicate that a number of fatality victims might have been revived through the intelligent and efficient use of the methods outlined in the *JAMA* articles.

To gain confidence in these rescue procedures, water safety personnel should understand why each step in the rescue procedure is used. To accomplish this they must first become familiar with the physiology of drowning.

Through experiments with dogs, it has been demonstrated that a definite sequence of events occurs during drowning. This same sequence is thought to occur in humans, with one further addition. Upon submersion the victim undergoes a stage of breathholding; he then involuntarily swallows large volumes of water. This in turn results immediately in vomiting.

The next stage is found in the human but not in the dog, and it is called laryngospasm.

Laryngospasm is the closing of the airway by the tonic contraction of the laryngeal muscles and is thought to be initiated by the tactile stimulus of water drops touching the mucous membrane of the larynx, which in turn sets off a characteristic reflex by way of the (sensory) superior laryngeal nerve. This is part of man's survival mechanism, preventing water from entering his lungs, but, after a sufficient period of asphyxia has existed at the neuromuscular synapses of these muscles, they relax, causing the airway to reopen. It is up to this stage, which should not be more than four minutes in duration, that the victim has suffered from acute asphyxiation with possibly a certain amount of vomitus obstructing the airway but nothing more.

It is with the beginning of the stage immediately following the release of the laryngospasm that various other phenomena occur, each of these depending upon the type of water (salt, fresh, or chlorinated) in which the person drowns.

Reprinted with permission from *Today's Health*, July 1965, Vol. 43, No. 7, pp. 46-48 and 66, published by the American Medical Association.

This stage, called the terminal gasp stage, results in the aspiration of water into the victim's lungs.

Aspiration of fresh water free from irritants demonstrated in experiments on dogs, using deuterium oxide tracers, that within two minutes after initiation of the terminal gasp stage, the blood stream was found to contain as much as 50 percent aspirated water. This hemodilution resulted in a lower concentration of sodium in the blood, which when combined with the now drastically low levels of oxygen in the body, produced the phenomenon called ventricular fibrillation.

Ventricular fibrillation is the irregular, spastic contractions of the ventricular muscles resulting in the loss of pumping action of the heart. Consequently, with loss of pumping action, the closing of the heart valves and the turbulence of the blood within the heart ceases, resulting in the total loss of heart sounds. Thus, this condition is impossible to distinguish from that of cardiac arrest even with the use of a stethoscope. It should therefore be kept in mind that the absence of heart sounds by the stethoscope does *not* mean that all cardiac activity has ceased.

In aspiration of salt water the principal variations in this type of drowning are: first, an elevated concentration of sodium in the blood due to passage of salt (sodium and chloride ions) through the alveolar membranes, and second, fulminating pulmonary edema, which is the swelling of the alveolar membranes caused by the accumulation of edema fluid within the lungs. Due to the increased thickness of the alveolar membrane in lungs with pulmonary edema, the ability of oxygen to pass across the alveolar membranes is greatly reduced.

In previous studies of aspiration of fresh water containing irritants, it was found that chlorinated water, such as occurs in swimming pools where free chlorine is added as a disinfectant, did not pass across the alveolar membranes of the lung and into the bloodstream as did clean, fresh water. Instead, a rapid and severe exudation into the lungs occurred, resulting in pulmonary edema. This is thought to be caused by the chemical irritation of chlorine upon the alveolar membranes of the lung.

Almost any chemical substance or particulate matter such as would occur in dirty water will be an irritant to the exceedingly delicate alveolar membrane. The resulting pulmonary edema (accumulation of fluid upon the alveolar membranes of the lung) and aspiration pneumonitis (the inflammation and swelling of the alveolar membranes due to irritating substances that have been aspirated) are the principal variations in this type of drowning. They also are thought to be the reason why aspirated fluid does not pass across the alveolar membranes into the bloodstream to any significant degree such as occurs in fresh water drowning. These findings, based on research, have been substantiated by at least one actual documented case of chlorinated water drowning reported in *JAMA*.

It is significant to note that, in both chlorinated and salt water aspiration cases, the level of sodium and chlorine within the bloodstream does not decrease to the critical degree that is seen in fresh water aspiration cases. Consequently, the danger of ventricular fibrillation occurring in the two former categories is very small.

Emphasis must be placed upon the need for a rapidly initiated and efficiently carried-out procedure. Through experiments on animals it was shown that within three to five minutes after the onset of asphyxia, the higher brain centers began to suffer damage, and that after eight minutes, the damage was irreparable. Consequently, the conservation of time in carrying out rescue procedures is of utmost importance. During approximately the first four minutes after submersion, the victim suffers from asphyxia with possibly some airway obstruction, but nothing more.

During this stage the victim has his greatest chance for survival, providing the proper means are used quickly and efficiently. If the victim remains submerged longer than this period of time, he enters the final stages, beginning with the release of the laryngospasm, resulting in aspiration of water into the lungs, and finally, death. It is not known how long this sequence takes, but it is certainly the most critical period of all.

It is during this period that every applicable rescue measure explained in this article must be utilized. In experiments on dogs, it was shown that mouth-to-mouth resuscitation was not enough to revive victims in this final period. It was also shown that intermittent positive pressure ventilation (resuscitator) with 100 percent oxygen revived a high percentage of the victims within this same critical period.

The addition of carbon dioxide to the oxygen was formerly advised in order to stimulate respiration. It is now believed that for purposes of resuscitation, oxygen should be used without added carbon dioxide. Whenever tissues are anoxic they contain an excess of carbon dioxide. Consequently, an added amount is not needed to stimulate the respiratory center of the brain.

The following procedure is designed for use in all three of the previously mentioned types of drowning. Not all the steps outlined need be used in every case, but rather their initiation is dictated by the individual victim.

When the victim is first reached, the rescuer should determine whether he still is breathing. Three signs of the body's lack of oxygen are unconsciousness, blue lips, and the rolling back of the eyes. If the victim is not breathing, or if his breathing efforts are too small to detect, the rescuer must immediately clear the mouth of any obstruction and begin mouth-to-mouth resuscitation.

This type of emergency resuscitation is recommended because of its superior ability to inflate the lungs over that of older methods. It also enables the rescuer to maintain an open air passage by holding the victim's head in a flexed position. And in cases where the laryngospasm is still present, it reopens the air passage by means of the blown air and results in the permanent relaxation of the laryngeal muscles.

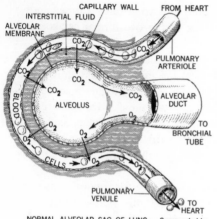

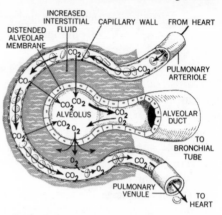

NORMAL ALVEOLAR SAC OF LUNG — Surrounded by capillary which picks up the oxygen and carries it throughout the body

ALVEOLAR SAC WITH PULMONARY EDEMA — NOTE: Reduced size of Alveolar Sac due to thickened Alveolar Membrane and Interstitial area. This results in a decrease in the amount of oxygen being able to pass into the blood stream.

As soon as the mechanical resuscitator becomes available it should replace the mouth-to-mouth method. This is necessary for a number of reasons. Through experiments on dogs it was found that within four minutes after submersion the victim's oxygen tension in the blood drops from 100 percent to approximately 10 percent or lower. Thus, the sooner his oxygen debt is replenished, the better will be his chances for revival. Due to the decreased effectiveness of the lungs for gas exchange in the presence of pulmonary edema, it is essential to use the method utilizing the greatest amount of oxygen.

It is easy to see that the mechanical resuscitator delivering 100 percent oxygen will fulfill this condition much better than mouth-to-mouth resuscitation, which delivers a little less than 20 percent oxygen. The value of this difference is evidenced in the previously mentioned findings that the mechanical intermittent positive pressure resuscitator, delivering 100 percent oxygen, was still able to revive victims in periods where mouth-to-mouth resuscitation was no longer effective.

Another piece of equipment of utmost importance in the rescue procedure is the stethoscope. This is a delicate instrument which is used to detect the slightest heart sounds of the drowning victim. If no heart sounds are detected, it can be assumed the heart is either in ventricular fibrillation or cardiac arrest. In either case, the treatment is the same — external cardiac massage.

It is most important that only a person who has been specially trained in external cardiac massage should attempt this procedure.

During external cardiac massage the victim's legs should be elevated at an angle of at least 60°. The subsequent decrease in blood flow into the legs due to gravity causes more of the vital oxygen carrying blood to flow to the brain, where the oxygen debt is much more critical.

This will reestablish and maintain circulation until the heart starts pumping by itself again, or in the case of ventricular fibrillation, until it can be defibrillated in the hospital. Due to the important roles the mechanical resuscitator and stethoscope play in the rescue procedure, it is of utmost importance that they are kept in a strategically located spot and are ready to be put into use immediately.

Upon the resumption of breathing efforts the victim should be supported by oxygen inhalation. This allows the victim to breathe on his own while being exposed to an environment of 100 percent oxygen. When the victim's breathing efforts become strong enough, he may be taken off 100 percent oxygen and allowed to breathe normal air again. The rescuer must be cautioned not to make this switch suddenly. Why? Such a rapid change often is quite distressing to the victim, who would suffer from an inadequate supply of oxygen.

Another variation in the drowning victim is the previously mentioned phenomenon of pulmonary edema. This may manifest itself within moments after the victim is brought up from the water. To the rescuer, pulmonary edema is observed as a frothy, blood-like fluid oozing from the victim's nose and mouth, especially during the exhalation phase of the breathing cycle. Due to appearance, it is sometimes mistakenly interpreted as simply broken blood vessels within the nose. In this situation the rescuer will again find the stethoscope of value, this time in determining whether pulmonary edema is present. If present, the stethoscope will transmit a rasping or congested sound within the lungs. Sometimes it is so severe and loud that heart sounds cannot be heard.

If pulmonary edema is indicated, it is of utmost necessity that the victim's airway be kept clear of this fluid by means of an aspirator. It may be wise to point out that portable units are commercially available which contain the aspirator assembly in combination with the resuscitator-inhalator assembly. The rescuer should place the aspirator suction tube (catheter) into the victim's throat by insertion through the nose rather than the mouth due to easier guidance and less chance of getting it stuck. Continuous aspiration is not necessary, but rather periodic aspiration as the accumulation of fluid dictates.

In addition to the above procedures, it is necessary to keep in mind the importance of conserving the victim's body heat during this critical period. This is done by covering the victim with a blanket as soon as he is brought from the water.

It must be emphasized that the rescuer's responsibility does not end with the victim's revival. Due to the critical strain the victim's body has undergone, and to such systemic alterations as hemodilution (a reduced ratio of blood cells to plasma), his condition may deteriorate within minutes after revival. He may again undergo ventricular fibrillation or respiratory arrest. Consequently, the rescuer must remain on the alert for untoward reactions until the victim is in the hands of a physician.

STAY-ALIVE RULES FOR SWIMMERS

Many drownings could be avoided if individuals would adhere to a few basic rules while swimming or engaging in water sports:

1. Learn to swim and relax in the water.
2. Never swim alone.
3. Do *not* swim when overly tired or when the water is extremely cold.
4. Do *not* overestimate your ability and endurance.
5. Swim at protected pools or beaches under the supervision of a trained lifeguard.
6. If a boat overturns, stay with it and don't try to swim a long distance to shore.
7. Never dive into unknown waters.
8. Try new activities only after learning the skills from qualified instructors.

Private pools are increasing rapidly in the United States. If you have a private pool, or use a neighbor's, observe some fundamentals of safety:

- Make certain the pool is kept clean and the water chemically purified.
- Walk, don't run, about the pool. Horseplay should be forbidden.
- Fence the pool and keep the gate locked to keep out small children.
- Keep handy rescue equipment, such as long poles and ring buoys.
- Keep bottles and glasses away from the concrete or metal pool deck.

When the Heart Stops

Paul W. Kearney

One day last May, Bertie Bish, 67, of Baltimore, crumpled in agony across his bed. His wife found him there. With a scream she ran to the telephone and dialed the fire department. "Please send an ambulance," she said. "My husband ..." Bertie Bish's heart was acting up again.

The ambulance, with crewman Hubert Cheek and Marvin Burkendine aboard, arrived several minutes later, siren moaning. By this time Bish was unconscious. His heart stopped beating. His face took on the bluish tinge of imminent death.

In any place but Baltimore, lay ambulancemen like Cheek and Burkendine would have been helpless to do anything except rush him to the hospital. Had a doctor been present he might have tried to restart the heart with a few hard blows of his fist on Bish's chest. Possibly forcing pure oxygen into the lungs might have started the heart pumping again. But the chances would have been slight.

The doctor might have performed a dramatic emergency operation: cut open Bish's chest and reached in to massage the heart with his hand (a procedure known to doctors as "rhythmical manual compression of the heart"). Such operations are performed almost every week. But even in skilled hands in a fully equipped hospital this is a measure fraught with risk. Most certainly it is not for firemen, policemen, or first-aiders.

But Bish was lucky. Only four days earlier the two Baltimore ambulance-men had been taught a new technique which promises to revolutionize the emergency treatment of cardiac arrest — a technique almost as simple in its way as in the first-aider's recently approved and widely publicized mouth-to-mouth breathing for starting respiration. Developed at Johns Hopkins Hospital, it is called "closed-chest heart massage." It requires no surgery, no equipment. It is applicable not only in a heart attack but in cardiac arrest from drowning, choking, electrical shock, chemical asphyxiation, shock from drug sensitization, or any other accident which causes the heart to come to a standstill. It can be used, reported its developers in the *Journal of the American Medical Association*, by anyone, anywhere. All that is needed are two hands.

To work on Bertie Bish, ambulancemen Cheek and Burkendine quickly stretched him flat on his back on the floor. Cheek knelt at Bish's side and tilted Bish's chin up and back, pointing it toward the ceiling, to keep his tongue from obstructing his windpipe. He then placed the heel of his right hand on the unconscious man's breastbone, in the center of the chest, over the heart. He put his left hand on top of his right. With a quick firm thrust he pushed down with both hands, hard enough to depress Bish's chest one inch. This would squeeze some of the blood out of the heart into the big arteries. Then Cheek lifted his hands, to let Bish's chest expand and let some of the blood from the big veins flow into the heart. He did this 70 times a minute: press . . . release . . . press . . . release.

Meanwhile, the second ambulanceman knelt at Bish's head and began mouth-to-mouth breathing, to force oxygen into Bish's lungs. This part of the technique must be foregone, of course, if the rescuer is working alone — the chest pressure provides some ventilation of the lungs anyway. But respiratory aid does tremendously increase the victim's chances of surviving with his brain undamaged from a lack of oxygen.

Cheek and Burkendine worked on Bish for only a minute before his pulse began a faint beat. After five minutes he had begun to breath without assistance. In the ambulance they gave him oxygen and Cheek continued the closed-chest massage right into the emergency room at the hospital, where doctors took over. Today Bertie Bish walks around Baltimore marveling at his experience — the first case of cardiac arrest on record to be snatched from death by trained first-aiders using closed-chest massage.

This lifesaving technique was developed by W.B. Kouwenhoven, Ph.D., a Johns Hopkins electrical engineer, with the help of others on the staff of the Johns Hopkins University School of Medicine. The doctors experimented with it on dogs for two years before attempting it on humans. Then one day a 35-year-old woman's heart stopped while she was undergoing surgery. The surgeon massaged her heart without opening her chest. After two minutes her pulse returned, and the surgeon went on with the operation.

On other occasions, the heart of a 12-year-old boy suddenly stopped while he was being given anesthesia. A 45-year-old man's heart stopped and he fell to the hospital floor while he was removing his clothing for an examination. An 80-year-old woman's heart stopped while she was undergoing surgery for cancer. In each case the doctors revived the patients with closed-chest massage. They brought back to life 14 of the first 20 cases they tried it on, or 70 percent. By mid-August they had used the technique successfully on 44 out of 56 more emergencies — a remarkable record when compared with the results of cutting open the chest to massage the heart directly, which even in hospitals has proved only about 40 percent effective.

As Johns Hopkins doctors are quick to point out, the figures aren't quite as optimistic as they seem. This is because, whatever the technique used, some resuscitated heart-arrest patients die, perhaps hours or days later, of the very thing that caused the original arrest. Yet the results still have been so impressive that last May Dr. Alfred Blalock, chief of surgery at the hospital, had the technique taught to the Baltimore fire department's ambulance service supervised by Captain Martin C. McMahon. Within three months, the ambulancemen revived six cases of heart standstill which had occurred on the street or in the victims' homes. Among them was one of their own firemen, a battalion chief, whose heart stopped after he was overcome by smoke while fighting a blaze. Now Captain McMahon is demonstrating the closed-chest massage technique to other ambulance and rescue squads.

To the men he is training, Captain McMahon stresses eight points:

1. Check for pulse — the easiest place to detect it is not in the wrist but in the throat, on either side of the windpipe near the collarbone. If no pulse is apparent, start working on chest massage at once. Don't waste seconds going for equipment or help. For the great peril of any heart or breathing arrest is anoxia — lack of a sufficient supply of oxygen, carried in the blood, to feed the brain. The brain is the most sensitive tissue of the body, and the results of oxygen starvation become irreversible within a few minutes — usually about three — after respiration or circulation is cut off. Hence a victim who survives belated treatment faces the possibility of extensive brain damage.

2. Lay the patient face up on a solid support, such as the floor or pavement; a bed or couch is too flexible.

3. Tilt the head back until the chin is practically pointing at the ceiling. If the head sags forward the patient may be asphyxiated while you work.

4. Kneel so you can use your weight in applying pressure. Place the heel of your right hand on the breastbone, with fingers spread and raised so that pressure is only on the breastbone, not on the ribs.

5. Place your left hand on top of the right and press vertically downward, firmly enough to depress the breastbone one to one-and-a-quarter inches. (With a child, use only one hand and relatively light pressure.) The chest of an adult, resistant when he is conscious, will be surprisingly flexible when he is unconscious.

6. Release the pressure immediately, lifting the hands slightly, then repeat in a cadence of 60 to 80 thrusts per minute, approximately the normal heart action.

7. The patient should be taken to the hospital as soon as possible. Even if apparently normal heartbeat and respiration have resumed, professional care will be needed.

8. Continue the closed-chest massage until you get professional medical aid, or right into the emergency room of the hospital. Continue too, if possible, the mouth-to-mouth breathing until someone arrives with a tank of oxygen to take over. If you are on your own and the victim shows no response, continue the massage until rigor mortis sets in.

Even trained and experienced medical men find it increasingly hard to say when a person is really dead beyond recall. Many of the old signs — like dilated eye pupils which won't contract under a bright light — are no longer considered valid. Thirteen years ago an eminent Cleveland surgeon set a heart to beating after 75 minutes of open-chest manipulation. Johns Hopkins doctors recently revived another cardiac-arrest victim after 105 minutes of closed-chest massage plus administration of oxygen. Sometimes, as the great physiologist Yandell Henderson of Yale once said: "The engine is merely stalled and needs to be cranked."

Closed-chest massage, in proper hands, may prove to be a highly useful crank to get the standstill heart moving again.

Cardiopulmonary Resuscitation

In May 1966, the work of an ad hoc Committee on Cardiopulmonary Resuscitation culminated in a Conference on Cardiopulmonary Resuscitation at the National Academy of Sciences-National Research Council (NAS-NRC). This study was undertaken in response to inquiries from the American National Red Cross and other national and federal agencies concerned with the need for standardized techniques of performance, training, and retraining requirements, and designation of the categories of persons to be taught mouth-to-mouth ventilation and external cardiac compression under present limitations on the supply of instructors. The ad hoc committee carefully reviewed and discussed these matters with representatives of over 30 national organizations attending the conference. The full proceedings of the conference will be published by the NAS-NRC. A summary of the recommendations of the ad hoc committee follows.

In November 1958, a Conference on Artificial Respiration was held at the National Academy of Sciences—National Research Council, and led to the publication in January 1959 of a "Statement on Emergency Artificial Respiration Without Adjunct Equipment." This statement unanimously endorsed the mouth-to-mouth and mouth-to-nose techniques of artificial respiration as the most practical methods of emergency ventilation without adjunctive equipment for an apneic person of any age. Since then, there has been worldwide acceptance and application of these techniques.

In July 1960, the clinical efficacy of an external manual technique for artificial circulation was reported. Since that time, well-documented experimental and clinical studies have established that the proper combination of artificial respiration and external cardiac compression can sustain a victim of sudden cardiac arrest for a reasonable period. Early experiences revealed both the benefits and the hazards of external cardiac compression and the need for its precise coordination with effective methods of artificial respiration by properly trained persons.

In an editorial in *Circulation* in September 1962 (1), closed-chest cardiopulmonary resuscitation was endorsed as a *medical* procedure. Subsequently, the method was reclassified as an *emergency* procedure in a second editorial in *Circulation* in May 1965 (2). This was endorsed by the American Heart Association, the American National Red Cross, the Industrial Medical Association, and the U.S. Public Health Service, which strongly recommended that the technique should be applied by "properly trained individuals of medical, dental, nursing and allied health professions and of rescue squads."

Statement by the Ad Hoc Committee on Cardiopulmonary Resuscitation of the Division of Medical Sciences, National Academy of Sciences-National Research Council. Reprinted from the *Journal of the American Medical Association*, 24 October 1966, Vol. 198, No. 4, pp. 373-379, with permission from the American Medical Association.

Since publication of the second editorial, the American Heart Association, the Public Health Service, and other organizations have inaugurated intensive training programs in cardiopulmonary resuscitation in response to the widespread interest and enthusiasm of highly motivated persons at all levels from first aid workers to professional medical personnel. Their experiences have indicated that clinical results vary widely and depend upon the exact technique taught, the effectiveness of training and periodic retraining, the personnel taught, the selection of cases, and numerous other factors. These considerations have guided the ad hoc Committee on Emergency Cardiopulmonary Resuscitation in formulating the following recommendations.

ABCD Steps

Emergency cardiopulmonary resuscitation involves the following steps:
A – *A*irway opened
B – *B*reathing restored
C – *C*irculation restored
D – *D*efinitive therapy
These should always be started as quickly as possible and always in the order shown. The recommended basic steps for performing the ABCs are shown in the Figure. Definitive therapy involves diagnosis, drugs, defibrillation (when indicated), and disposition. These definitive procedures are restricted to physicians or to members of allied health professions and paramedical personnel under medical direction. They are beyond the scope of this statement, which will be restricted to the ABCs of emergency cardiopulmonary resuscitation.

Exhaled-Air Ventilation (Mouth-to-Mouth Ventilation; Mouth-to-Nose Ventilation)

A and B are the basic steps of artificial ventilation and should always be applied first in emergency resuscitation. They constitute first aid measures which can be performed under almost any circumstances without adjunctive equipment or help from another person and regardless of the cause of the apnea.

The most important single factor contributing to successful resuscitation is immediate opening of the airway. This is most easily and quickly accomplished by maximum backward tilt of the head. Sometimes an unconscious patient will be saved by this simple maneuver, which reestablishes an open airway and allows spontaneous breathing to resume. With the patient supine, the rescuer places one hand behind the patient's neck and the other on his forehead. He then lifts the neck and tilts the head backward. This stretches the neck and lifts the tongue away from the back of the throat, thereby relieving this anatomical obstruction of the airway. The head should be maintained in this position at all times.

Obvious foreign material in the mouth or throat should be removed immediately with the fingers or by any other means possible.

If the patient does not resume spontaneous breathing after his head has been tilted backward, immediately begin artificial ventilation by either the mouth-to-mouth or the mouth-to-nose method. The first blowing effort will determine whether or not any obstruction exists. For mouth-to-mouth ventilation the patient's head is maintained in a position of maximum backward tilt with one hand behind the neck. In the unconscious patient this usually allows the mouth to drop open. The nostrils are pinched together with the thumb and index finger of the other hand. The rescuer then opens his mouth widely, takes a deep breath, makes a tight seal with his mouth around the patient's mouth, and blows in about twice the amount the patient normally breathes. He then removes his mouth and allows the patient to exhale passively. This cycle is repeated approximately 12 times per minute. Adequate ventilation is ensured on every breath by (a) seeing the chest rise and fall, (b) feeling resistance of the lungs as they expand, and (c) hearing the air escape during exhalation.

Mouth-to-nose ventilation can be used if it is impossible to open the patient's mouth, if it is impossible to ventilate through his mouth, if his mouth is seriously injured, if it is difficult to achieve a tight seal, or if the rescuer prefers the nasal route. For this technique the rescuer keeps the patient's head tilted back with one hand and uses the other hand to push the patient's lower jaw closed and seal his lips. He then takes a deep breath, seals his lips around the patient's nose, and blows in until he sees the patient's chest rise. He then removes his mouth, allows the patient to exhale passively, and repeats the cycle 12 times per minute. When mouth-to-nose ventilation is employed it may be necessary to open the patient's mouth during exhalation, if this can be done, to allow the air to escape.

Occasionally, there may be incomplete opening of the air passages even with properly performed "head-tilt." In such cases, further opening of the air passages can be achieved by displacing the patient's mandible forward so that his lower teeth are in front of his upper teeth, and by simultaneously holding his mouth open. This may be accomplished (a) by grasping the mandible between the thumb and index finger and lifting, or (b) by placing the fingers behind the angles of the lower jaw and pushing it forward.

A and B are performed in essentially the same way for children, except that for infants and small children the rescuer covers the patient's mouth and nose with his mouth and blows gently, using less volume to inflate the lungs. Babies require only small puffs of air from the rescuer's cheeks. The rate of inflation should be 20 to 30 times per minute. The neck of an infant is so pliable that forceful backward tilting of the head may obstruct breathing passages; therefore, the tilted position should not be exaggerated.

The presence of a foreign body should be strongly suspected if the rescuer is unable to inflate the lungs after proper head tilt and foward displacement of the mandible. The first blowing effort will determine whether or not any obstruction exists. An adult patient with this problem should be rolled onto his side quickly and firm blows delivered over his spine between the shoulder blades in an attempt to dislodge the obstruction. The rescuer's fingers should then be swept through the patient's mouth to remove such material. Then exhaled-air ventilation should be resumed quickly. Sometimes, slow forceful breaths can be used to bypass a partial airway obstruction and inflate the lungs. A small child with an obstructive foreign body in the airway should be picked up quickly and inverted over the rescuer's forearm while firm blows are delivered over the spine between the shoulder blades. Then quickly resume ventilation.

Exhaled-air ventilation frequently causes distension of the stomach. This occurs often in children, and is not uncommon in adults. It is most likely to occur when excessive pressures are used for inflation or if the airway is not clear. Slight gastric distension may be disregarded. However, marked and easily discernible distension of the stomach may be deleterious because it promotes regurgitation, reduces lung volume by elevating the diaphragm, and may initiate vagal reflexes. Obvious gross distension should be relieved whenever possible. In the unconscious patient this can be accomplished by using one hand to exert moderate pressure over the patient's epigastrium between the umbilicus and the rib cage. If a second rescuer is available he can prevent recurrence of gastric distension by maintaining moderate pressure in this area. Special attention should be directed to lowering the patient's head or turning it to one side, or both, during this maneuver, to avoid aspiration of gastric contents.

No adjuncts are required for effective exhaled-air ventilation, and such devices usually do not increase the effectiveness of the method. Accordingly, there should be no delays caused by seeking such equipment or by putting it into use. If desired, a clean cloth or handkerchief can be used to cover the patient's mouth or nose, to overcome the esthetic and hygienic objections to direct oral contact. When available and properly employed, various devices (masks, tubes, airways) may be useful for professional medical and paramedical personnel.

Every effort should be made to teach exhaled-air methods of artificial ventilation to as many members of the general populace as possible. The ad hoc committee urgently recommends that steps be taken to ensure training of the entire population from the fifth-grade level upward, by schools, clubs, local and national first aid groups, and medical, paramedical, and rescue organizations. Training should be according to the technique described above and in accordance with the training standards of the American National Red Cross. For optimum results it should include such media as lectures, demonstrations, posters, slides, and movies. Actual practice on life-like training manikins increases the efficiency of performance and is recommended, although it is not essential for satisfactory performance. When used, such manikins should provide obstruction of the airway when the head is not tilted back maximally, allow mouth-to-mouth and mouth-to-nose ventilation, and result in rise of the chest when the lungs are inflated.

Alternative Methods of Artificial Ventilation

Regardless of the method used, the preservation of an open airway is essential. This can best be done by ensuring continued extension of the head and neck and forward displacement of the lower jaw. Some unconscious victims will be saved simply by establishing an open airway and permitting spontaneous breathing to resume.

The ad hoc committee recommends exhaled-air ventilation as being unequivocally superior to all manual methods since it provides for control of the airway at all times, allows immediate assessment of airway obstruction, monitors ventilation on a breath-to-breath basis, and provides more actual ventilation than any of the manual methods. Furthermore, external cardiac compression cannot be used effectively in conjunction with manual methods. Manual methods should be used only in special circumstances that make it impossible or ill-advised to use exhaled-air methods. These include crushing facial injuries, conditions where the head is trapped, situations on the pole-top, etc.

Those rescuers who cannot or will not use the exhaled-air techniques should use a manual method. No one manual method can be recommended as being unequivocally superior to the others. Some techniques are more effective than others, depending on the circumstances, and the rescuer should not be limited to the use of a single manual method for all cases.

The supine Chest-Pressure Arm-Lift method (Silvester) is generally preferred, especially when used with an improvised support under the shoulders. This tends to maintain an open airway because of backward tilt of the patient's head when he is in the supine position. Turning his head to one side is also useful in that it reduces the hazard of aspiration of vomitus. When a second rescuer is available he should endeavor to maintain proper head and neck position or forward displacement of the mandible, or both. When possible, the patient should be inclined to promote drainage of the lungs, with his head lower than his body.

The push-pull prone manual methods – Back-Pressure Arm-Lift (Holger Nielsen) and Back-Pressure Hip-Lift – can provide some ventilation, but the possibility of airway obstruction is always present, even with assistance of a second rescuer to keep the patient's head extended and to displace his mandible forward. The advantage claimed, that gravity alone will provide an open airway by causing forward displacement of the mandible with use of the prone position, cannot be substantiated in the unconscious patient. Furthermore, the prone position restricts movement of the thorax and abdomen, thereby restricting ventilatory volume.

Cardiopulmonary Resuscitation (CPR)
(Heart-Lung Resuscitation [HLR])

After three to five effective lung inflations, the carotid pulse should be checked. The operator maintains head-tilt with one hand; with index and middle fingers of the other hand he gently locates the larynx, and, after sliding laterally with the fingers flat, he palpates the carotid area. The pulse should be "felt," not "compressed." If apnea persists and there is unconsciousness, death-like appearance, and absence of carotid pulse, external cardiac compression should be started. External cardiac compression consists of the application of rhythmic pressure over the lower half of the sternum. This compresses the heart and produces a pulsatile artificial circulation because the heart lies almost in the middle of the chest between the lower sternum and the spine. When properly performed, it can produce systolic blood-pressure peaks of over 100 mm Hg, with a mean blood pressure of 40 to 50 mm Hg in the carotid artery and carotid arterial blood flow of up to 35% of normal.

External cardiac compression must always be accompanied by artificial ventilation. Compression of the sternum produces some artificial ventilation but not enough for adequate oxygenation of the blood. For this reason artificial ventilation must be used whenever external cardiac compression is used.

Effective external cardiac compression requires sufficient pressure (80 to 120 pounds) to depress the patient's lower sternum 1½ to 2 inches in an adult; the rate should be once a second. For external cardiac compression to be effective, the patient must be on a firm surface. If he is in bed, a board or improvised support should be placed under his back, but compression must not be delayed for that purpose. The rescuer stations himself at the side of the patient and places only the heel of one hand over the lower half of the sternum. Care must be exercised not to place the hand over the tip or xiphoid process of the sternum which extends down over the upper abdomen. He places his other hand on top of the first one and then rocks forward so that his shoulders are almost directly above the patient's chest. Keeping his arms straight, he exerts adequate pressure almost vertically downward to move the lower sternum 1½ to 2 inches in an adult. The preferred rate of 60 per minute is usually rapid enough to maintain blood flow and slow enough to allow cardiac refill; it is also practical in that it avoids fatigue and facilitates timing on the basis of one compression per second. The compressions should be regular, smooth, and uninterrupted, with compression and relaxation being of equal duration. Under no circumstance should compression be interrupted for more than five seconds.

When there are two rescuers, optimum ventilation and circulation are achieved by quickly "interposing" one inflation after each five chest compressions without any pause in compressions (5:1 ratio). One rescuer performs external cardiac compression while the other one remains at the patient's head, keeps it tilted back, and continues exhaled-air ventilation. Interposing the breaths without any pause in compressions is important, since every interruption in cardiac compression results in a drop of blood flow and blood pressure to zero. When there is only one rescuer he must perform both artificial ventilation and artificial circulation using a 15:2 ratio, i.e., two quick lung inflations after each 15 chest compressions.

The technique is similar for children, except that the heel of only one hand is used for small children and only the tips of the index and middle fingers for babies. The ventricles of infants and small children lie higher in the chest and the external pressure should be exerted over the midsternum. The danger of lacerating the liver is greater in children because of the smallness and pliability of the chest and the higher position of the liver under the lower sternum and xiphoid. The force of compression should be sufficient to move the sternum about one fifth of the distance from the front to the back of the chest. In infants up to 1 year old this results in adequate blood-pressure peaks with 10 to 15 lb of pressure. Children up to 6 years old require 20 to 25 lb of pressure. The compression rate should be about 100 times per minute with breaths interposed after each five compressions. For infants and small children, backward tilt of the head arches the back off the horizontal. Firm support for external cardiac compression can be provided if the rescuer slips one hand beneath the patient's back while using the other hand to compress his chest. An alternate method for small infants is to encircle the chest with the hands and compress the midsternum with both thumbs.

The reaction of the pupils should be checked during cardiopulmonary resuscitation, since it provides one of the best clews to the overall status of the patient. A pupil which constricts when exposed to light indicates adequate oxygenation and blood flow to the brain. If the pupils remain widely dilated and do not react to light, serious brain damage is imminent or has occurred. Dilated but reactive pupils are less ominous. Normal pupillary reactions may be altered by the administration of drugs.

Periodic palpation of the carotid or femoral pulse should be employed to check the effectiveness of external cardiac compression or the return of a spontaneous effective heartbeat. The carotid pulse is more meaningful and more practical to use than the femoral or radial pulse.

Complications can occur from the use of cardiopulmonary resuscitation. These include fracture of the ribs and sternum, laceration of the liver, and fat emboli. They can be minimized by careful attention to details of performance. Several important admonitions for proper performance of this technique are as follows: (a) Never compress over the xiphoid process at the tip of the sternum.

This bony prominence extends down over the abdomen and pressure on it may cause laceration of the liver, which can be lethal. (b) Never let your fingers touch the patient's ribs when compressing. Keep just the heel of your hand in the middle of the patient's chest over the lower half of his sternum. (c) Never use sudden or jerking movements to compress the chest. The action should be smooth, regular, and uninterrupted, with 50% of the cycle compression and 50% relaxation. (d) Never compress the abdomen and the chest simultaneously. This traps the liver and may cause it to rupture.

There must always be a maximum sense of urgency in starting external cardiopulmonary resuscitation. The outstanding advantage of this technique is that it permits the earliest possible treatment of cardiac arrest without any equipment and by other than professional medical personnel. The time between recognition of need and start of treatment should be measured in seconds.

A maximum sense of urgency must continue throughout the resuscitation procedures. Never interrupt heart-lung resuscitation for more than five seconds at a time for any purpose — moving the patient, changing rescuers, checking the pulse or electrocardiogram, injecting drugs, intubating the airway, applying mechanical devices, etc. With practice and attention to details this can usually be accomplished. The concept that the state of urgency no longer exists once artificial ventilation and artificial circulation have been established is completely erroneous. The longer it is necessary to continue cardiopulmonary resuscitation the less likely it is to succeed. Even under optimum circumstances deterioration is progressive during heart-lung resuscitation, and the sense of urgency must be preserved until all efforts are abandoned.

External cardiopulmonary resuscitation may be ineffective when certain conditions exist. These include crushing injuries of the chest, internal thoracic injuries, cardiac tamponade, tension pneumothorax, or severe emphysema with enlargement and fixation of the rib cage. If it can be determined that any of these conditions is present and if a physician is present with the necessary skill, equipment, and facilities in a hospital or other medical installation, he should open the chest and perform internal cardiac compression in conjunction with artificial ventilation. A decision to use the internal method or cardiac compression may also be made under the proper circumstances by physicians who doubt the efficacy of the closed-chest method in particular cases or after prolonged application.

Cardiopulmonary resuscitation should not be started when it is known or can be determined with a degree of certainty that cardiac arrest has persisted for more than five or six minutes (probably longer in drowning). If there is a question of the exact duration of the arrest, the patient should be given the benefit of the doubt and resuscitation started. If cardiopulmonary resuscitation is started in the absence of a physician, it should be continued until one is available to assume responsibility. Cardiopulmonary resuscitation is not indicated in a patient who is known to be in the terminal stage of an incurable condition.

The decision to stop cardiopulmonary resuscitation is a medical one and depends upon an assessment of the cerebral and cardiovascular status. The best criteria of adequate cerebral circulation are the reaction of the pupils, the level of consciousness, movement, and spontaneous respiration. Deep unconsciousness, absence of spontaneous respiration, and fixed, dilated pupils for 15 to 30 minutes are indicative of cerebral death and further resuscitative efforts are usually futile. Cardiac death may be assumed when there is no return of electrocardiographic activity after one hour of continuous cardiopulmonary support. In children, resuscitative efforts should be continued for longer periods than in adults since recovery has been seen even after prolonged unconsciousness.

Training in Cardiopulmonary Resuscitation

Heart-lung resuscitation is an emergency procedure which requires special ability in the recognition of cardiac arrest and special training in its performance. All training programs should adhere to the standards of the American Heart Association as detailed in its training manual. Experience has shown that, in addition to lectures, demonstrations, slides, and films, actual practice in both the ventilatory and the circulatory components of cardiopulmonary resuscitation is required on life-like manikins. An initial course in cardiopulmonary resuscitation should require a minimum of three hours of training for small groups of students and should include sufficient supervised, intensive manikin practice for every student to become proficient in detecting the presence or absence of the pulse and in performance of the individual steps and sequence of exhaled-air ventilation, external cardiac compression, and the combination of the two. Courses for instructors in cardiopulmonary resuscitation should, whenever possible, include practice in all of the ABCDs on experimental animals.

Retraining or refresher courses which include manikin practice are required for all personnel. The exact frequency of such retraining may need to be regulated on the basis of the professional skill and experience of particular groups. However, the retraining requirements suggested at present for other than medical groups are twice the first year and annually thereafter.

All physicians, dentists, osteopaths, nurses, inhalation therapists, and rescue personnel should be carefully trained in heart-lung resuscitation. Training should be provided by either physicians or instructors who have had special instructor courses in cardiopulmonary resuscitation under such organized programs as those of the American Heart Association and the Public Health Service.

Cardiopulmonary resuscitation should not be taught to the general public at the present time. However, the committee recognizes that carefully controlled pilot projects should be carried out with highly motivated, select groups of lay personnel in order to determine the feasibility and effectiveness of such programs. Furthermore, instruction in heart-lung resuscitation for the general public cannot be inaugurated until sufficient numbers of trained instructors are available.

The committee also recognizes the desirability of certification in cardiopulmonary resuscitation set up under agencies with officially approved training-retraining programs. Such certification should indicate satisfactory completion of an approved cardiopulmonary resuscitation training course, or satisfactory training to serve as an instructor in cardiopulmonary resuscitation.

Use of Mechanical Equipment in Conjunction With Cardiopulmonary Resuscitation

Attempts at reoxygenation of the lungs by exhaled-air methods or via mask should always precede attempts at tracheal intubation. Adequate lung inflations, interposed between external cardiac compressions, require high pharyngeal pressures which promote gastric distension. Therefore, the trachea should be intubated as soon as possible by trained personnel.

Manually operated self-inflating bag-valve-mask units are recommended, since their use by trained personnel permits assessment and correction of ventilation volumes, airway obstruction, mask leak and gastric insufflation, and proper timing of inflations without interference with external cardiac compressions.

The highest possible inhaled oxygen concentration should be provided as soon as possible. By the use of a self-inflating bag-valve-mask unit, inhaled oxygen concentrations of over 50% can be obtained only by attaching to the intake valve a reservoir tube with a capacity equal to the tidal volume and an oxygen inflow rate of at least the minute volume. By attaching a demand valve to the bag intake, 100% inhaled oxygen concentration can be obtained.

Conventional pressure-cycled automatic ventilators or resuscitators are not recommended for use in conjunction with external cardiac compression because effective cardiac compression triggers termination of the inflation cycle prematurely, producing shallow and insufficient ventilation. The inflation flow rates of this type of equipment are usually inadequate.

Oxygen-powered manually triggered ventilation devices are acceptable if they can provide instantaneous flow rates of 1 liter/sec, or more, for adults. A safety-valve release pressure of about 50 cm of water should be provided. Ideally, they should permit the use of 100% oxygen and support of airway and mask with both hands. For use on infants and small children, specialized mechanical breathing devices producing lower flow rates are required.

External cardiac compression machines are adjuncts which may be used when prolonged resuscitation or transportation of the patient is required. They should be designed to approximate performance of the manual method. Their design should facilitate head-tilt and quick application of the machine, and minimize the danger of accidental malpositioning of the plunger during use. If automatic ventilation is also provided, it should be programmed to inflate the lungs after every fifth compression without a pause. When inflation is by face mask, gastric distension may occur and is an indication for gastric decompression and tracheal intubation.

External cardiac compression must always be started with the manual method first. When mechanical devices are used, one rescuer must always remain at the patient's head to monitor plunger action and ventilation, to check the pulse and pupils, and to support head-tilt and mask-fit manually unless the trachea is intubated.

Members of the ad hoc committee: Warren H. Cole, MD, *Chairman*, University of Illinois Medical Center, Chicago; Larry H. Birch, MD, Butterworth Hospital, Grand Rapids, Mich; James O. Elam, MD, Kansas City (Mo) General Hospital; Archer S. Gordon, MD, Lovelace Clinic and Foundation, Albuquerque, NM; James R. Jude, MD, University of Miami (Fla) School of Medicine; Peter Safar, MD, University of Pittsburgh School of Medicine; Leonard Scherlis, MD, University of Maryland School of Medicine, Baltimore; *Ex Officio Members:* Robert L. Flynn, MD, US Public Health Service, Washington, DC; Robert M. Oswald, American National Red Cross, Washington, DC; J. Keith Thwaites, American Heart Association, New York; Leroy D. Vandam, MD, Peter Bent Brigham Hospital, Boston; Sam F. Seeley, MD, NAS-NRC staff, Washington, DC.

This study was supported by the Division of Health Mobilization, Public Health Service, contract PH86-65-104, and by the American National Red Cross.

REFERENCES

1. "The Closed-Chest Method of Cardiopulmonary Resuscitation: Benefits and Hazards." *Circulation* 26 (September 1962): 324.
2. "The Closed-Chest Method of Cardiopulmonary Resuscitation: Revised Statement." *Circulation* 31 (May 1965): 641.

Cardiopulmonary (Heart-Lung) Resuscitation

Asphyxia

When breathing stops for any reason a condition results which is known as asphyxia.

The physiological causes of asphyxia may include lack of stimulation of the respiratory center in the brain, paralysis of the respiratory center, and inability of the blood to absorb oxygen from the lungs or to effect the normal exchange of gases in the body tissues.

When it is due to physical causes, it may be spoken of as suffocation. In asphyxia resulting from physical causes, the lungs are deprived of air because of stoppage of the air passages mechanically. Such causes may include water in the air passages, as in drowning; foreign body in the air passages; tumor in the air passages; swelling of the mucous membrane in the nose and throat, following inhalation of live steam or an irritating gas; constriction around the neck, compressing the windpipe; and the lack of oxygen from any cause. The most frequent causes of stopping of breathing are drowning, electrical shock, and gas poisoning. Asphyxia may be present also in victims of shock or collapse, of extreme exposure to heat or cold, and chemical poisoning. Whatever the cause of asphyxia, death will result unless breathing is started quickly. A few seconds' delay in starting artifical respiration may lead to fatal result.

Symptoms of Asphyxia

1. Cyanosis (blueness of skin).
2. Breathing stopped.
3. Shallow breathing in some cases of poisoning.

Treatment of Asphyxia

The first thing to do in treatment is to remove the cause of the asphyxia or to remove the patient from the cause. Then administer artificial respiration. Later treat as for shock. In some cases artificial respiration can be administered while the patient is being removed from the cause to more suitable surroundings. The treatment for shock can often be started while artificial respiration is being administered.

The patient's mouth should be cleared of any obstruction, such as chewing

Reprinted from *Coastguard*, April 1969, a publication of the Department of Transportation, United States Coast Guard.

gum, tobacco, false teeth, or mucus, so that there is no interference with the entrance into and escape of air from the lungs.

Artifical respiration should be started immediately. Every moment or delay is serious. It should be continued at least 4 hours without interruption, until normal breathing is established or until the patient is pronounced dead by a medical officer.

Not infrequently the patient, after a temporary recovery of respiration, stops breathing again. The patient must be watched and if natural breathing stops, artificial respiration should be resumed at once. Perform artificial respiration gently and at the proper rate. Roughness may injure the patient.

General Principles of Manual Artificial Respiration

Time is of prime importance. Seconds count. Do not take time to move the victim to a more satisfactory place; begin at once, i.e., while victim is still in water as in case of drowning victim. Do not delay resuscitation to loosen clothes, warm the victim, or apply stimulants. These are secondary to the main purpose of getting air into the victim's lungs.

Begin artificial respiration and continue it rhythmically and without interruption until spontaneous breathing starts or the victim is pronounced dead by a medical officer.

As soon as the victim is breathing by himself, or when additional help is available, see that the clothing is loosened (or removed, if wet) and that the patient is kept warm, but do not interrupt the rhythmic artificial respiration to accomplish these measures.

If the victim begins to breathe on his own, adjust your timing to assist him. Do not fight his attempts to breathe. Synchronize your efforts with his.

Do not wait for a mechanical resuscitator; but when one is available, use it as an inhalator. The important advantages of good mechanical resuscitators are that they are not fatiguing, and can furnish 100 percent oxygen. Because a resuscitator need only be applied to the patient's face, it can be used when physical manipulation of the body is impossible or would be harmful, as during surgical procedures, in patients with extensive burns, broken vertebrae, ribs and arms, for victims trapped under debris of excavations, or under overturned vehicles, and during transportation of the victim. Furthermore, some resuscitators signal when the airway is obstructed and provide an aspirator.

Remember, it is all-important that artificial respiration, when needed, be started quickly. A check should be made to ascertain that the tongue or foreign objects are not obstructing the passages. A smooth rhythm in performing artificial respiration is desirable, but split-second timing is not essential. Shock should receive adequate attention, and the subject should remain recumbent after resuscitation until seen by a physician or until recovery seems assured.

Cardiopulmonary Resuscitation

Definition: An emergency first aid procedure that combines *artificial respiration* with *artificial circulation*.

The best rescue technique for artificial respiration is mouth-to-mouth breathing.

The best rescue technique for artificial circulation is external cardiac massage.

Mouth-to-Mouth Breathing .

+   . Cardiopulmonary Resuscitation

External Cardiac Massage   .

Mouth-to-mouth breathing should be started at once in any case where breathing has ceased. This may be due to any one of many causes including:

1. Drowning.
2. Suffocation.
3. Electrocution.
4. Poisonous gases.
5. Heart attack.

Only *after* mouth-to-mouth breathing has been started and *after* it has been determined that the heart has stopped should external cardiac massage be started and combined with mouth-to-mouth breathing to give cardiopulmonary resuscitation.

Many cases will be encountered in which the person has stopped breathing but whose heart is still going and these cases require only mouth-to-mouth breathing.

Cardiopulmonary resuscitation must be started without delay. You have only 4-5 minutes in which to initiate this rescue technique. After that time irreparable damage has occurred in the vital organs. Therefore, you DO NOT leave the victim to summon aid. If another person is present send him for help, but start resuscitation immediately. Don't waste time moving the victim except when there is actual physical danger present. Any delay might be the difference between success and failure.

Cardiopulmonary Resuscitation Technique

The following techniques will govern cardiopulmonary resuscitation procedures . . .:

A. *Mouth-to-Mouth Breathing*

1. This is ALWAYS started first and then the necessity for external cardiac massage is determined.

2. Place victim on his back (Figure 1).

3. Kneel beside head (Figure 2).

4. *Clear mouth and air passages of foreign objects, i.e., chewing gum, dentures, seaweed (drowning victims), etc.* (Figure 7).

5. Place one hand under victim's neck (Figure 3).

6. Place other hand on victim's forehead so that thumb and forefinger can close the nose (Figure 4).

7. Lift gently with hand under neck while pushing down with hand on forehead. This will extend the neck and open the air passages in the vast majority of cases (Figure 5).

8. Take a deep breath (about twice the normal), open your mouth widely, place your mouth over victim's mouth and blow (Figure 6).

9. Watch for victim's chest to rise. As soon as this happens remove your mouth from victim's and let natural recoil expire from victim.

10. Repeat 12-14 times a minute for adults, 18-20 for children and infants.

11. If chest does not rise one or more of the following conditions exist and must be corrected.

    a. Airleak.

        (1) Make sure that there is airtight seal between your mouth and the victim's and that seal on victim's nose is secure.

    b. Airway obstruction (more likely).

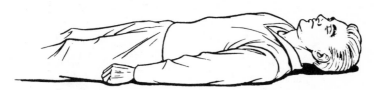

Figure 1. Victim on firm surface.

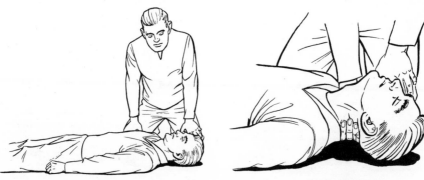

Figure 2. Rescuer in position.   Figure 3. Hand under neck.

(1) Insert finger into victim's mouth and remove any foreign bodies (false teeth, etc.), vomit and/or blood clots (Figure 7).

c. If chest still fails to rise, remove hand from neck, insert thumb into mouth and grab lower jawbone (mandible) between thumb and fingers and lift jawbone upward holding it in this position while you continue to perform mouth-to-mouth breathing (Figure 8).

12. In children and infants a lesser amount of air is necessary. In infants the amount of air that can be held in your cheeks may be sufficient. However, if your mouth is removed quickly as soon as the chest begins to rise no damage will be done.

13. Mouth-to-nose breathing may be carried out using much the same technique except, of course, the victim's mouth is held closed while your mouth is placed over the victim's nose (Figure 9).

14. If you would hesitate to place your mouth over the victim's, satisfactory mouth-to-mouth breathing may be carried out through a handkerchief. Airways and tubes should not be used by Coast Guard personnel. Not only are they dangerous when used by untrained personnel but usually are not available when such an emergency arises.

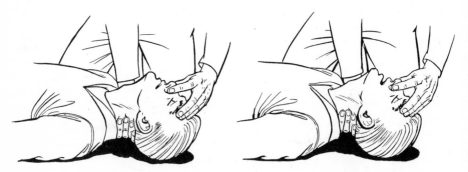

Figure 4. Hand on forehead. Nose closed.   Figure 5. Neck extended.

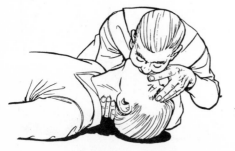
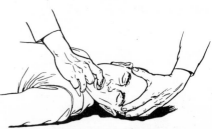

Figure 6. Actual inflation.   Figure 7. Cleaning air passages.

B. External Cardiac Massage

1. After mouth-to-mouth breathing has been instituted with 5-6 quick breaths, and only then, check to see if external cardiac massage should be started.

    a. It is needed only if the heart has stopped.

    b. In many cases the institution of mouth-to-mouth breathing will be sufficient to cause resumption of the heartbeat.

2. Check for a pulse.

    a. The best pulse to check is the carotid in the neck. This is a large artery lying close to the surface on either side of the Adam's apple (Figure 10). Practice feeling your own.

3. Check the pupils.

    a. If the pupil is widely dilated and doesn't contract (get smaller) when light hits it, then blood flow to the brain is insufficient.

4. If there is no pulse and/or the pupil is widely dilated and doesn't contract start external cardiac massage.

5. Locate notch at top of breastbone (Figure 11).

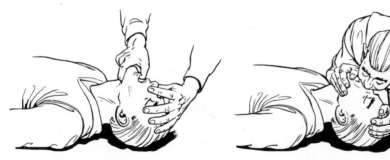

Figure 8. Elevation of jaw.   Figure 9. Mouth to nose.

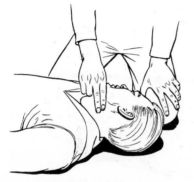
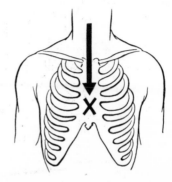

Figure 10. Carotid pulse.   Figure 11. Sketch of sternum.

6. Locate lower end of breastbone (Figure 11).

7. Place heel of one hand over lower one-third of breastbone (Figure 11 "X") and other hand on top of first (Figure 12).

8. Compress breastbone against backbone by exerting downward pressure on hands with the weight of your upper body.

9. Pressure is then released quickly. This cycle is repeated 60-80 times per minute in adults, 80-100 in children.

10. Breastbone should move 1½ to 2 inches in adults. Children's chests are not as strong and external cardiac massage in infants can be done with 2 fingers while in older children up to age 10 one hand usually suffices.

11. Fingers should be kept *away* from the ribs to avoid fractures (Figure 12).

12. Check pulse frequently to see if heart has restarted.

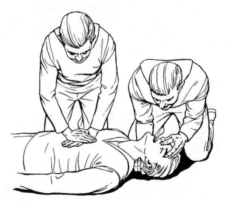

Figure 12. Position of hands.

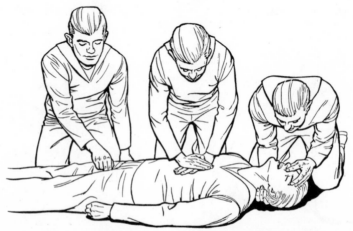

Figure 13. Cardiopulmonary resuscitation by three rescuers.

Some Additional Factors in Cardiopulmonary Resuscitation

1. If three rescuers are available after someone has been sent for help they should be utilized as follows (Figure 13):
    a. One to administer mouth-to-mouth breathing.
    b. One to administer external cardiac massage.
    c. One to monitor the pulse preferably in the groin (to check adequacy of massage).
        (1) Rhythm may be adjusted by giving 4 to 5 strokes on the breastbone followed by one lung inflation. Stroke, stroke, stroke, stroke, breath, etc.
        (2) Timing may be estimated by counting 1001 (one thousand and one) for each stroke which closely approximates one second.

2. If two rescuers are present —
    a. One administers mouth-to-mouth breathing.
    b. One administers external cardiac massage.

3. If only one rescuer is present he must of necessity administer both mouth-to-mouth breathing and external cardiac massage. This can be managed by interrupting external cardiac massage every 30 beats to give 5 or 6 lung inflations.

4. Stomach may become distended with air. This is especially true if airway is not clear. It is not dangerous and can be remedied by applying pressure over the stomach with the palm of one hand. This expels the air but may also lead to regurgitation of the stomach contents so you must be ready to turn the head to one side and clean out mouth with fingers or cloth (Figure 7).

5. Cardiopulmonary resuscitation, once started, must be continued until spontaneous breathing and heartbeat occur or until victim is turned over to a physician. In many cases this will mean that the procedure must be continued while victim is being transported to medical facilities.

6. In cases of submersion (apparent drowning) do not attempt to drain fluid from lungs. If possible have head lower than body, but even this is not essential.

7. If more than 5 minutes have passed since the heart stopped then external cardiac massage should not be used. If the time interval is unknown then give the victim the benefit of the doubt and start massage.

Summary

When

Cardiopulmonary resuscitation should be started at once in any case where breathing and the heart have stopped. If only breathing has stopped use mouth-to-mouth breathing. Don't waste time seeking help or equipment. Begin at once.

Who

YOU. By following the simple preceding instructions any [adult]. . .can perform cardiopulmonary resuscitation. Almost 70 percent of successful rescues are accomplished by persons at the scene of the accident. This could be you.

Where

Resuscitation should be performed where the victim is found. Don't waste valuable time moving him, finding special equipment, seeking additional help, getting him out of the water, etc. It is necessary to move him only if there is actual physical danger present.

How

Follow these simple instructions:
1. Put victim on firm surface, face up.
2. Start mouth-to-mouth breathing.
3. Check for heart beat, pulses, dilation of pupils.
4. If heart has stopped begin external cardiac massage.
5. Continue cardiopulmonary resuscitation until a physician takes over or until victim's breathing and heart beat have started again.

General Rules and Information

The general rules outlined below are set forth as a guide to determine the proper course of action under various conditions and to establish effective coordination with appropriate local organizations. . . .

There is no substitute for thorough training, advance planning and good judgment. A specific rule for each case cannot be made. Decisions as to whether a patient should be turned over to another team arriving on the scene, or as to the best choice of method under a given set of circumstances, must be made by the person in charge.

In any case, when a . . . team using a manual method gives way to a resuscitator team, the person in charge of the resuscitator team becomes responsible for the patient. However, the first aid personnel shall continue to render every assistance they are able to furnish for bringing the resuscitation to a successful conclusion.

The mechanical resuscitator, sometimes referred to as the pulmotor, which is not generally furnished to a first-aider, is an apparatus that supplies oxygen or a mixture of oxygen and carbon dioxide, while inspiration and expiration are being induced by the application of alternating pressure. Although this equipment has its place when manned by skilled personnel, it is possible that it may operate as a hazard rather than a help if inaptly handled. Most resuscitators can be set up to operate as simple inhalators. Risks connected with the use of the pressure feature of the resuscitators can thus usually be avoided simply by using the resuscitator as an inhalator. It should be noted, however, that the inhalator *will not* do the job by itself. There must be a mechanical movement of air to facilitate resuscitation. This is best accomplished by the mouth-to-mouth method using the inhalator after the person has started to breathe by himself or where the person has difficulty breathing, i.e., a patient with broken ribs.

Treatment of Shock

When the patient revives, he should be kept under close observation for 48 hours even though he apparently feels all right. He should not be permitted to exert himself in any way.

The fundamental factors in the prevention and treatment of shock are heat, position, and stimulants.

A. Heat

1. Preserve body heat.
    a. Protect from exposure to cold.
    b. Remove wet clothing and dry the patient.
    c. Wrap the patient loosely in dry blankets.
2. Application of external heat.
    a. Artificial means of warming (hot bricks, water bottles) are not indicated routinely because it encourages the undesirable dilatation of surface vessels and may cause a further depletion of blood fluids through sweating and, of course, the warming agents may burn the casualty.
    b. Should artificial heat be deemed necessary, care should be taken to:
        (1) Test the object used for applying heat by holding against the cheek or elbow for half a minute.
        (2) Wrap in a layer of cloth or paper before applying to patient.
    c. Methods:
        (1) Hot water bottles
        (2) Chemical heating pads
        (3) Glass jars and bottles containing warm water.
        (4) Warmed bricks
        (5) Electrical heating pads
    d. Regions where external heat may be applied:
        (1) Soles of feet
        (2) Between the thighs
        (3) Along the sides of the body
        (4) Over the abdomen if not uncomfortable to the patient.

B. Position

1. Place the body in such a position so that gravity will help the blood flow to the brain and heart.

    a. Lay the patient on his back with the head low.

        (1) This can be accomplished by raising the foot of the bed, cot, bench, or litter at least 12 inches higher than the head unless the patient complains of discomfort. Then either follow (2) below or let the patient remain lying flat and quiet.

        (2) If on a flat surface and other means are not available, elevate the feet, legs, and thighs.

C. Stimulants

Do not attempt to make an unconscious person drink. If conscious, give small quantities at a time.

1. Aromatic spirits of ammonia — a teaspoonful in half a glass of water — is one of the most satisfactory stimulants. This can be repeated every 30 minutes as needed.

2. Coffee and tea both contain the drug caffeine, which is an excellent stimulant. Give the coffee or tea as hot as can be comfortably taken. A cupful may be given every 30 minutes as needed.

3. Hot milk, or even hot water, has some stimulating effect, due to the heat.

4. An inhalation stimulant, such as an ammonia ampule or aromatic spirits of ammonia on a handkerchief, may be placed near the patient's nose in cases in which the patient is not conscious. The one administering the stimulant should always test it on himself first.

5. Whiskey should not usually be given.

Treatment of Poisoning Emergencies

First Aid for Poisoning

Brent Q. Hafen, Ph.D.

The increased availability of common household and commercial cleaners, drugs, and other chemical substances that have potential toxic effects on the human body has increased the common first aid emergency of poisoning. This is particularly true among children. Because of the widespread availability of toxic substances and increased incidence of poisoning, it has become obvious that speed and effective action in even the simplest of poisoning cases is of utmost importance.

In recent years many poison control centers have been opened throughout the U.S. These centers are constantly updating their information on the latest available antidotes and treatment for new toxic substances, including common household cleaners as well as the most potent drugs. These centers are especially organized and set up to handle all types of poisoning cases and usually maintain a detailed file of information so they will be able to give immediate and specific emergency treatment.

Many communities now have poison control centers. Most of these are in connection with a hospital. It is suggested that you check to see if your community has a poison control center, and list its phone number in a place where it could be quickly found in case of a poisoning emergency. This should be done before the emergency arises.

In the advent of a poison emergency, you should call one of the poison control centers for assistance or get the victim to the center as soon as possible. If there are no centers available in the particular area of emergency, the victim should then be taken to a hospital emergency room after adequate and immediate first aid assistance has been rendered.

If poisoning is suspected, first aid measures must be prompt and as specific as possible. Immediate general first aid treatment should be aimed toward preventing the absorption of the poison and combating the effects of the poison that has already been absorbed.

Symptoms of Poisoning

The following is a suggested outline for general first aid treatment of poisoning. First there would be reason to suspect that a poison has been taken when any of the following symptoms or behavior are present: severe nausea, vomiting, diarrhea, collapse or convulsions, muscle twitching, delirium, unconsciousness, signs of fear or panic, signs of burns about the mouth or on the skin, agitation, restlessness or drowsiness, unusual flushing or exceptional pallor, and pain, especially sudden pain without previous signs. Sometimes the pain or burning sensation will be localized in the throat area. Also a characteristic odor might be detected on the breath, or there may be discoloration of the lips and mouth.

What To Do Until Medical Help Arrives.

Once it is suspected that poisoning has occurred, speed is essential. If possible, one person should administer first aid while another calls a physician or poison control center.

Answers to the following questions when contacting the physician for help may greatly enhance the speed with which the physician is able to take the necessary treatment steps once your emergency first aid measures have been rendered. What type and how much of the poison was taken? Is there any evidence of burns about the lips and mouth? Are the gums discolored? Is there any skin rash or discoloration? Is there an odor on the breath? Does the rate of respiration seem to be unusual? Does there seem to be any cyanosis? If vomiting has occurred, what is the general odor and appearance of the vomitus? Does there seem to be any muscular twitching or delerium or difficulty in speech if the victim is conscious, or does he seem to be in a coma or a stupor? Does his temperature seem to be subnormal or elevated? A first-aider should not spend a great deal of time trying to determine the answers to these questions before sending for help; however, a general recall of some of the things noticed while adminstering first aid might be of great help to the physician. It would also be important to retain the container, if one is found, from which the poison was taken, and also a specimen of the vomitus, if easily and quickly available.

The order in which you decide to render first aid measures may be as important as things that you actually do. It is obvious that the first thing which should be done is to send for a doctor, take the person to a doctor, or get someone else to call the doctor while you perform the basic first aid procedures. There are a few general principles that are applicable for any case of poisoning – these are important and should be learned. One, immediately call a doctor, arrange to get the victim to a doctor, or send someone for help. Two, remove the source of poison or the victim from the poison. This might mean diluting and/or inducing vomiting. Three, counteract the poison if at all possible with some suitable antidote. This is not always possible as a first aid measure and quite often would be the doctor's responsibility. Four, attempt to counteract the effect of the poison to some degree by treating for shock and other symptoms that may occur. The order in which these principles are applied would not be the same in all cases. Sometimes the removal of the poison as the immediate first aid measure would be more important than calling the doctor, although these things can sometimes be done simultaneously if additional first aid help is available.

Ingested Poisons

The following first aid measures should be followed for a poison that has been ingested. The first thing that should be done is dilute the poison. This will delay absorption and also aid in washing out or emptying the stomach if it is necessary to induce vomiting. Water is the safest and most available treatment for the victim to swallow. If readily obtainable, milk, egg whites, and similar substances should also be used to delay absorption and help protect the lining of the digestive tract.

Next, vomiting should be induced unless the victim is in a coma, unconscious, in convulsions, has swallowed some type of petroleum product such as kerosene, lighter fluid, gasoline, etc., or has swallowed a corrosive poison. If a petroleum product has been ingested, administer two ounces of vegetable oil. If burns or stains exist around the victim's mouth and lips, this would be indicative that the poison was a corrosive and again vomiting should not be induced. This type of poison has the symptoms of severe pain, burning sensation in the mouth and throat, and sometimes vomiting. The acid and acid-like corrosives are substances such as toilet bowl cleaners, nitric acid, silver nitrate, rust removers, and sodium acid sulfate. Alkali corrosives are substances such as drain cleaners or the hydroxide lyes, sodium carbonates such as washing sodas, ammonia water, and the household bleaches or sodium hydrochloride.

If the poison was any of the foregoing acid-type corrosives or acids such as carbolic acid, or phenyl and hydrochloric acid, vomiting should *not* be induced but the individual should be given some form of a neutralizer immediately, such as magnesium chalk or limewater. Also, milk, olive or any vegetable oil, or raw egg white should be given to protect the lining of the digestive tract. The individual should then be kept warm and treated for shock. The strong alkali corrosives, again, can cause destructive action. If the person has swallowed a strong alkali, do *not* induce vomiting but give a weak acid such as lemon juice or vinegar in order to neutralize the alkali. Also give him milk, olive or vegetable oil, melted butter, or raw egg white to help protect the lining of the digestive tract.

Inducing Vomiting

In cases other than the aforementioned, vomiting should be induced by giving 1 teaspoon baking soda to a glass of warm water; soap suds, a fairly strong solution; salt water — a teaspoon salt to a glass warm water; mustard water — a half teaspoon powdered mustard to a glass of warm water; alum water — a a quarter teaspoon powdered alum to a glass of warm water; or by tickling the back of the throat.

Antidotes

After the stomach has been emptied by vomiting, it is necessary to administer the proper antidote if it is immediately available. You should never take time, however, to find the antidote before emptying and washing out the stomach. There are three different types of antidotes that are often used in the emergency treatment of poisoning cases. Two of these would possibly be used by a first-aider. The first is referred to as a physical antidote and is one that mixes with or envelopes the poison, prevents it from being absorbed, and may also sooth and protect the tissues of the digestive tract. Common first aid substances of this type would include milk, egg whites, olive oil, starch, barley water, mashed potatoes. The second type is a chemical antidote and is one that reacts on the poison and neutralizes it. Common first aid chemical antidotes would be substances such as milk of magnesia or baking soda or magnesium oxide that are chemical antidotes for acids, whereas lemon juice, grapefruit juice, and vinegar are weak acids that can be used to neutralize strong bases. A third is a physiologic antidote. This is an antidote that produces the opposite effect from that of the poison. These are usually in the form of drugs that would be administered by the physician in the treatment of poisoning.

A commercial version of a universal antidote is often recommended. This consists of one part of tannic acid, one part of magnesium oxide and two parts activated charcoal. It is suggested that the tannic acid part of the universal antidote precipitates heavy metals, the magnesium oxide neutralizes any acidic substances, and the activated charcoal acts as an absorbent.

Further, the American Red Cross has suggested that if a commercial mixture of the universal antidote is not available that this can be substituted by one part of strong tea, one part of milk of magnesia, and two parts of crumpled burnt toast. The commercial version of the universal antidote does seem to have some value because of the absorptive quality of charcoal — even though the absorption of poison is lessened when the charcoal is combined with tannic acid and magnesium oxide. However, the homemade version of the universal antidote, consisting of burnt toast (charcoal), tea (acid), and milk of magnesia (alkali), is of little value because the type of charcoal provided by burnt toast is not the kind that absorbs poison.

Summary

(1) Diluting substances in cases where the individual is not convulsing or unconscious should be given immediately to delay absorption. These can be milk, egg white, beaten whole egg, or some type of flour in suspension, or starch or even mashed potatoes in water. Of course, if nothing else is available, water should be used to dilute the poison and reduce the possible effects on the tissues in the digestive system. (2) Vomiting should be induced by giving one of the previously mentioned emetics or by tickling the back of the throat with the finger or the blunt end of a spoon, with the exception of corrosive products and petroleum products. (3) A specific antidote should then be administered if it is

available. (4) Treat for shock in all cases of poisoning, conserve body heat, and administer artificial respiration if breathing stops. (5) When contacting the poison control center or the physician the following information would be helpful:

When the poison was taken, the age and sex and approximate size of the victim, what poison was taken or the trade name of the product, how much was taken, type of symptoms that are being exhibited by the victim, and also what you have done in the way of first aid measures.

The doctor and/or the poison control center should be notified by a second person if that individual is available while you are administering first aid. If you are alone, you need to exercise judgment and do whatever seems most urgent in that particular case. While seeking medical assistance if the victim is vomiting, for example, the individual should be placed face down with his head lower than his hips so that the vomitus cannot enter the lungs which might cause further damage or even perhaps suffocation.

Poisons on the Skin

For poison or chemical burns on the skin, the American Medical Association suggests the following first aid: immediately drench the skin with running water (shower, hose, faucet) and wash rapidly (and in some cases remove clothing) to reduce extent of poison absorption and possible injury.

For chemical burns (except by yellow phosphorus): immediately wash with running water and cover with loosely applied clean cloth. Avoid ointments, greases, powders, and drugs in any form. Treat for shock, keep victim warm, and reassure him until the physician arrives.

Inhaled Poisons

For inhaled poisons such as gas fumes, smoke, etc., the American Medical Association suggests the following:

(1) Carry or drag victim to fresh air immediately (do not let him walk). (2) Open all doors and windows. (3) Loosen all tight clothing. (4) Apply artificial respiration if breathing has stopped or is irregular. (5) Keep victim warm, prevent chilling (wrap victim in blanket if necessary). (6) Keep victim as quiet as possible. (7) If victim is having convulsions, keep him lying down in a semidark room and avoid jarring or noise. (8) Be careful not to become a victim yourself by exposure to the same poison. (9) Never give alcohol in any form.

Drug Poisoning

Drug availability and drug taking has increased tremendously in the past decade in our country. Ours has become a drug-taking society where many different kinds of drugs are used for a variety of purposes. Drugs are substances used to diagnose, treat, or prevent illnesses or substances that are used to modify body function in one way or another. They are often used to restore health, lessen pain, induce calmness, increase energy, create euphoria, induce sleep or alertness, and for a variety of other reasons. Some you swallow, some you drink, some are inhaled, and others are injected. Many of the drugs available today in the United States are for legitimate use in the practice of medicine. However, many of them are also subject to abuse, and there are other drugs that are not legally available on the market that are available illegally. There is also a long list of drugs and chemicals with no known medical use but with potent capacity to alter feelings and behavior. All of these drugs, whether they are used medically or otherwise, have toxic potential in the human body. With the increased availability and use of drugs in our country we have naturally seen an increase in drug poisoning, accidental and also in suicide cases. Because of this a first-aider should have some insight into and understanding of the various types of drug poisoning, of the types of symptoms that are manifested in specific drug groups and of the kind of first aid that can be rendered to alleviate a potentially dangerous and perhaps a life-threatening situation. For the purposes of this article we will discuss the drugs that are most commonly used and present the greatest threat to health and life with suggested emergency procedures for drug overdose. We will discuss these in three groups: the stimulants, the depressants, and the hallucinogens.

Stimulants

The stimulants are drugs that have a stimulating effect on the central nervous system. Those of greatest potential danger would be the amphetamines and cocaine. The amphetamines represent a group of drugs which exert a stimulating action of the cerebral cortex of the central nervous system. Examples of these drugs are benzedrine and dexedrine or dexoamphetamine and methamphetamine. These drugs are best known for their ability to combat fatigue and sleepiness. They are also quite often used to curb the appetite and thus have played a role in weight reduction. Applied externally to nasal membrane, amphetamines also have a constricting effect on blood vessels and were previously used in commercial products — nasal sprays and inhalants.

Amphetamines are known to people by various slang terms such as pep pills, wake ups, co-pilots, bennies, etc.

Cocaine is a natural drug which was used in the past as a local anesthetic. It has little medical use today. Cocaine is often referred to as "coke" or "snow" in slang terms. Cocaine is also a strong stimulant with action on the cerebral cortex. The amphetamines and cocaine may be taken orally or by injection. Cocaine is also inhaled in powder form. Common reactions of drug abuse or overdose from amphetamines and cocaine would be the following types of symptoms: irritability, tension, agitation, tremor, feeling of panic, and with large repeated doses, perhaps hallucinations and mental confusion. Reduction of fatigue, excitability, euphoria, talkativeness, enlarged pupils, heavy perspiration, loss of appetite are also very common. The abuser of cocaine often has feelings of great mental and physical prowess with feelings of courage and invincibility. More serious side effects would include abnormal heart rhythms, nausea, vomiting, sweating, and abdominal cramps. In serious cases there is often a drug type psychosis with delusions and hallucinations.

The victim of an overdose of amphetamines or cocaine is in need of calm, efficient help. This type of an individual should be given the assistance afforded and suggested in the section of this book that discusses psychological first aid and reducing environmental stimuli. Body temperature and an open airway should be maintained in all cases. It would be helpful to dilute with water or milk and then to induce vomiting if large doses of the drug were taken recently and orally. The person should then be taken to an emergency facility.

Depressant Drugs

The depressant drugs are those which have a depressant effect on the central nervous system and tend to calm activity and excitement and often promote sleep. One of the most common depressants, the barbiturates, are drugs which are derived from barbituric acid. These drugs are usually used in liquids, tablets, capsules, and sometimes other forms. Barbiturates are known to drug abusers as barbs, candy, goof balls, yellow jackets, red birds, red devils, inks, reds, blues, rainbows, and by various other slang terms, usually describing the appearance and nature of the form the drug comes in. These drugs include secanol, nembutal, and phenobarbital. The barbiturates are commonly used for sedation or to induce sleep. Overdoses, particularly when taken in conjunction with alcohol, may result in unconsciousness and death unless proper medical treatment is given immediately. The combination of alcohol and barbiturates produces an effect referred to as potentiation, where the effects of each drug is potentiated or increased by the action and effect of the two drugs in combination. Tranquilizers are other common depressants which are used to relieve mental tension and anxiety and relax muscles without producing sleep or seriously affecting mental and physical capacity. The more common ones would be meprobamate or diazapam. The typical signs and symptoms of abuse or overdose from these two types of depressants would be euphoria, impaired judgment, slurred speech, staggering, loss of balance and falling, a quarrelsome disposition and, with larger doses, sleep induction, perhaps leading in excessive doses to coma with the danger of death.

Another group of depressant drugs, the natural narcotics, are those derived from the opium poppy. These include drugs like morphine, codeine, and heroin.

Slang terms such as "horse," "smack," and "scag" are often used to describe heroin. These narcotics are often used medically for an analgesic or pain relief effect as well as for the depression of the cough reflex center in the brain, particularly in the case of codeine. Typical signs and symptoms of overuse of these drugs include constipation, loss of appetite, temporary impotency or sterility, dulling of the senses, a feeling or sense of well-being or euphoria, and a stupor which may lead to a coma and perhaps death.

One of the most common depressant drugs found in drug overdose problems is that of alcohol. Alcohol has very limited therapeutic value and is only of current interest because of its prevalent social use and abuse. Contrary to popular belief, alcohol does not stimulate the central nervous system but exerts a continuous depression upon it. If sufficient alcohol is ingested, anesthesis may be produced. Signs and symptoms of acute alcohol intoxication and overuse are well-known and include stupor, cold and clammy skin, slow respiration, low body temperature.

Ordinarily the condition requires no treatment other than sleep and passage of time; however, if the person is excited or in a state of coma, the following first aid should be attempted. (1) Send for medical help. (2) If the person is excited, take care to be calm and respectful. This type of individual should be given assistance as discussed in the section on psychological first aid. (3) If the person is unconscious, try to arouse him, if possible, and give him salt water, mustard water, soapy water, or similar emetic. If the person cannot be aroused, do not induce vomiting but seek medical help. (4) If the person's respiration becomes very shallow, employ artifical respiration.

In summary, then, we find that in the category of depressant drugs the most commonly abused drugs that lead to possible emergency situations are the barbiturates, the opiates, tranquilizers, and alcohol. In general, they depress mental activity and body functions. Excessive doses lead to loss of consciousness, low blood pressure, diminished respiration, and insufficient oxygen in the blood and other tissues. Sometimes the victim is able and willing to tell what he has taken. Sometimes the information is revealed through a container or a suicide note. If a person has taken a large or unknown dosage of a depressant durg, even though he is alert, severe depression may be delayed for several hours. By telephone a person should get advice from a physician or a poison control center. If a depressant drug has been taken recently by mouth, diluting and inducing vomiting may be helpful if the person is conscious. The most life-threatening situations occur with depressant overdoses of barbiturates and heroin. The danger is that of increasing stupor and cardiorespiratory collapse. In these cases it is imperative that the victim be taken to a physician or hospital as soon as possible, while maintaining body temperature and an open airway and giving artificial respiration if needed.

Hallucinogenic Drugs

Few drugs produce such a wide variety of effects as do the hallucinogens. Individual reaction is influenced by the personality of the subject, the setting in which the drug is taken, and the expectations of the individual taking the drug. The hallucinogenic drugs that most commonly produce emergency first aid situations are LSD (which is commonly referred to as acid), peyote or the more refined mescaline, psilocybin, and STP. Some of the other substances that may produce hallucinogenic effects include marihuana, DMT, DET, nutmeg, and even some types of morning glory seeds. Common symptoms from the abuse of the hallucinogens may include a distortion or intensification of the user's sense perception (visual and auditory), a lessening of his ability to discriminate between fact and fantasy, disproportional judgments of direction, distance, and objectivity, dilated pupils, eyes often extremely sensitive to light, and restlessness and sleeplessness. The mental effects are usually unpredictable, ranging from illusions, exhilaration, withdrawal, rapid mood swings, and self-destructive behavior to sheer panic. Some cases may include dizziness, headache, chilliness or heat flashes, and nausea. These types of drugs are potentially dangerous. Prolonged psychotic episodes characterized by hallucinations, anxiety, depression, suicide attempts, paranoia, and confusion have been known to be produced by such drugs. The physical effects are seldom a serious threat. However, a bad experience may result in fear and panic. This person needs a nonthreatening environment where he is being comforted and reassured. Someone should be with him at all times in quiet, safe surroundings. If he becomes frightened and starts to describe frightening sensations or images, his attention should be subtly diverted to something more pleasant. It is often helpful to reorient the person by describing the true situation without distortion. Other concepts discussed in the section on psychological first aid may be helpful. The victim should be taken to a physician or a hospital as soon as possible.

Curious Toddlers Fall Victims to Poison Accidents

Barbara Springer

What's one man's medicine could be another's poison . . . especially if that other person is a child.

Children, particularly two- and three-year-olds, are extremely curious — touching and tasting everything reachable. If there's any possible way to examine a tempting object — even if it's atop the refrigerator, on the top shelf of the medicine cabinet or in a purse or dresser drawer — a toddler probably will find a way.

This "toddler age" is a perfect stage for accidental poisonings. Another peak period is early adolescence, but, according to Dr. Anthony R. Temple, chief pediatric resident and a research fellow in clinical pharmacology and toxicology at the University of Utah Medical Center, such medicinal poisonings are rarely accidental. They're usually suicide attempts.

Aspirin Accidents

The most common poison is that great American cure-all, aspirin. According to the National Clearinghouse for Poison Control Centers, aspirin accounts for 19 percent of all accidental medicine poisonings. All medicines account for 53.4 percent of the poisonings.

The next largest category is cleaning and polishing agents, 14.5 percent. This group includes soaps, cleaners, bleach, lye, liquid polish and wax.

The major increase in child poisonings, though, is not an accidental overdose but a therapeutic overdose. "And this really bothers me," Dr. Temple stressed. "The child will get an overdose of medication from his parents. For example, they will give medicine without a physician's advice, or several family members will administer medicine without checking with each other."

Difficult To Diagnose

And therapeutic overdoses usually are more difficult to diagnose. They're even very easy to miss, Dr. Temple said, especially if the child has been sick a long time, the poisoning could come about gradually.

Surprisingly, for 90 percent of all poisons there is no antidote. Hence the ingested poison usually is either diluted or vomiting is induced, or both.

When someone is poisoned, the first thing to do is to immediately phone your physician, police, hospital or poison control center (there's one at the

Reprinted with permission from the *Salt Lake Tribune*, 5 May 1971, p. 8C.

university). Tell briefly and clearly what poison or medication has been taken, and, if you know, how much. Ask what to do until help arrives. (And when you take the person to the hospital or physician, bring along the bottle or container. It's valuable in diagnosis).

Incidences when vomiting should be induced are when the child has swallowed alcohol, camphor, DDT, food poisoning, iron compounds, laxatives, mushrooms and vitamin compounds.

To induce vomiting, Dr. Temple recommended one tablespoon of syrup of ipecac (non-prescription). Or you can give one teaspoon of dry mustard mixed with ½-cup water, or glass of warm water, or place the end of a blunt object at the back of the victim's throat.

Do not, however, make the child vomit if he is unconscious or having fits, has swallowed a poison which was a strong corrosive (such as lye, strong acid, drain cleaner), or has swallowed a poison containing kerosene, gasoline or petroleum distillates, like lighter fluid. Vomiting, in these instances, could cause further destructive damage to the stomach, intestines, esophagus tube.

To dilute the poison, so it won't be absorbed as rapidly into the blood stream and intestines, there are several possibilities. Dr. Temple particularly advocates giving one tablespoon of activated charcoal, it acts like a sponge, mixed with water. Several glasses of milk or water also would work.

There are several exceptions, though, to these methods of retarding absorption. If the poison is an acid, dilute it by mixing one tablespoon of milk of magnesia with one cup of water. If it's an alkali or alkaline substance (such as lye, ammonia, chlorine bleach, drain cleaner, detergents), give fruit juice or vinegar. And for petroleum distillates, dilute with milk or water and then give four tablespoons of vegetable oil. After diluting, get the patient immediately to the hospital.

Occurrence of Accidents

And if you don't know what your child (or an adult) has swallowed, "it's best to take him immediately to a doctor, or to a hospital emergency room," Dr. Temple stressed. "Even a half-hour delay could be dangerous."

When do most such accidental poisonings occur?

A recent study conducted by a medical team at the Karolinska Institute in Stockholm, Sweden, found that of 600 cases examined, at least one parent was at home in about three-fourths of the incidents. Most occurred in the kitchen, and usually when the child was left alone for only a short time. The peak time periods were between 11 a.m. and noon and between 4 and 6 p.m. — times when the child is getting hungry and is most apt to eat anything which looks like food, or anything which looks drinkable in a bottle.

Since a parent cannot be at the child's side every second, accidents can only be prevented by making it impossible for the child to harm himself. The place of storage of all potentially dangerous products must be both locked with a key and sufficiently high to be out of easy reach of the child. And never put dangerous products in containers which ordinarily are used for eating or drinking. To a child or even an adult, a bottle in the refrigerator or anywhere else means something to drink.

And Dr. Temple feels it would be "a particularly good practice if all medication were labeled (name and dosage), unless specified." The current practice, however, is, for the most part, not to so label medication unless specified. This policy, though, is changing.

The terrible tragedy is that the number of such poisoning accidents is increasing every year. In fact, nearly two million children are endangered by accidental poisoning annually in the nation; the deaths may run into the thousands. And some authorities regard the figures as only the tip of the iceberg, for many cases are either never reported or not diagnosed.

However, with simple precautions, proper knowledge and the two non-prescription emergency medicines (syrup of ipecac and activated charcoal), parents can protect their children from becoming one of the statistics.

Poison Antidote and Drug Counterdose Chart

DO THIS FIRST

- Send for a doctor— immediately.
- Keep the patient warm.
- Determine if the patient has taken
  - (1) A POISON
  - (2) AN OVERDOSE
- While waiting for physician, give appropriate counterdose below.
- But do not force any liquids on the patient — if he is unconscious.

- And do not induce vomiting if patient is having convulsions.

To Find The Correct Counterdose

- In one of the lists printed at right, find substance causing the trouble.
- Next to that substance is a number. This refers to counterdose bearing same number in the section below.

Keep all poisons and medicines out of reach of children

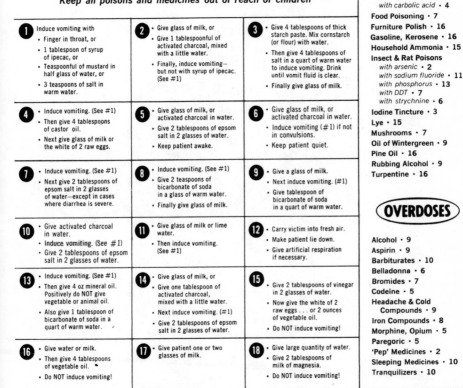

1 Induce vomiting with
- Finger in throat, or
- 1 tablespoon syrup of ipecac, or
- Teaspoonful of mustard in half glass of water, or
- 3 teaspoons of salt in warm water.

2
- Give glass of milk, or
- Give 1 tablespoonful of activated charcoal, mixed with a little water.
- Finally, induce vomiting— but not with syrup of ipecac. (See #1)

3
- Give 4 tablespoons of thick starch paste. Mix cornstarch (or flour) with water.
- Then give 4 tablespoons of salt in a quart of warm water to induce vomiting. Drink until vomit fluid is clear.
- Finally give glass of milk.

4
- Induce vomiting. (See #1)
- Then give 4 tablespoons of castor oil.
- Next give glass of milk or the white of 2 raw eggs.

5
- Give glass of milk, or activated charcoal.
- Give 2 tablespoons of epsom salt in 2 glasses of water.
- Keep patient awake.

6
- Give glass of milk, or activated charcoal in water.
- Induce vomiting (#1) if not in convulsions.
- Keep patient quiet.

7
- Induce vomiting. (See #1)
- Next give 2 tablespoons of epsom salt in 2 glasses of water—except in cases where diarrhea is severe.

8
- Induce vomiting. (See #1)
- Give 2 teaspoons of bicarbonate of soda in a glass of warm water.
- Finally give glass of milk.

9
- Give a glass of milk.
- Next induce vomiting. (#1)
- Give tablespoon of bicarbonate of soda in a quart of warm water.

10
- Give activated charcoal in water.
- Induce vomiting. (See #1)
- Give 2 tablespoons of epsom salt in 2 glasses of water.

11
- Give glass of milk or lime water.
- Then induce vomiting. (See #1)

12
- Carry victim into fresh air.
- Make patient lie down.
- Give artificial respiration if necessary.

13
- Induce vomiting. (See #1)
- Then give 4 oz mineral oil. Positively do NOT give vegetable or animal oil.
- Also give 1 tablespoon of bicarbonate of soda in a quart of warm water.

14
- Give glass of milk, or
- Give one tablespoon of activated charcoal, mixed with a little water.
- Next induce vomiting. (#1)
- Give 2 tablespoons of epsom salt in 2 glasses of water.

15
- Give 2 tablespoons of vinegar in 2 glasses of water.
- Now give the white of 2 raw eggs . . . or 2 ounces of vegetable oil.
- Do NOT induce vomiting!

16
- Give water or milk.
- Then give 4 tablespoons of vegetable oil.
- Do NOT induce vomiting!

17
- Give patient one or two glasses of milk.

18
- Give large quantity of water.
- Give 2 tablespoons of milk of magnesia.
- Do NOT induce vomiting!

POISONS

Acids · 18
Bichloride of Mercury · 14
Camphor · 1
Carbon Monoxide · 12
Chlorine Bleach · 17
Detergents · 17
Disinfectant
  with chlorine · 17
  with carbolic acid · 4
Food Poisoning · 7
Furniture Polish · 16
Gasoline, Kerosene · 16
Household Ammonia · 15
Insect & Rat Poisons
  with arsenic · 2
  with sodium fluoride · 11
  with phosphorus · 13
  with DDT · 7
  with strychnine · 6
Iodine Tincture · 3
Lye · 15
Mushrooms · 7
Oil of Wintergreen · 9
Pine Oil · 16
Rubbing Alcohol · 9
Turpentine · 16

OVERDOSES

Alcohol · 9
Aspirin · 9
Barbiturates · 10
Belladonna · 6
Bromides · 7
Codeine · 5
Headache & Cold
  Compounds · 9
Iron Compounds · 8
Morphine, Opium · 5
Paregoric · 5
'Pep' Medicines · 2
Sleeping Medicines · 10
Tranquilizers · 10

Reprinted with permission from *American Druggist*, 1970.

Commonly Abused Drugs — What You Should Know About Them

Name	Description	How taken	Initial effects	Long-term effects
Amphetamines (Benzedrine, Dexedrine, Methedrine)	Stimulants.	Swallowed, injected.	Agitation, talkativeness, insomnia, anorexia lasting 4-8 hours.	Possibility of infection, weight loss, high blood pressure, schizophrenic-like reaction. Psychological and physiological dependence.
Barbiturates (Amytal, Butisol, Nembutal, Pheno-barbital, Seconal, Tuinal)	Depressants. Made from barbituric acid.	Swallowed, injected.	Slurred speech, staggering and confusion, mood shifts lasting 4-8 hours.	Allergic reactions, convulsions Allergic reactions, convulsions, coma, death. Psychological and physiological dependence.
Cocaine (methylester of benzoylecgonine)	Stimulant. Made from leaves of cocoa bush.	Sniffed, swallowed, injected.	Excitation, loss of sense of time, exaggerated reflexes lasting a few minutes-4 hours.	Vertigo, confusion, exhaustion, convulsions, paralysis of respiratory center. Psychological dependence.
Codeine (methylmorphine)	Depressant. Weakest derivative of opium.	Swallowed.	Drowsiness, difficulty concentrating, dulled perceptions lasting about 4 hours.	Psychological and physiological dependence.
DMT (dimethyl-tryptamine)	Hallucinogen. Synthetic derivative of dimethyl-tryptamine.	Swallowed, injected, smoked.	Exhilaration, excitation lasting ½-4 hours.	Possible chromosome damage. Psychological dependence.
Heroin (diacetylmorphine)	Depressant. Synthetic alkaoid formed from morphine.	Injected, sniffed.	Euphoria, drowsiness and confusion lasting 4-8 hours.	Exposure to infection, chronic constipation, malnutrition, respiratory arrest. Psychological and physiological dependence.

Name	Description	How taken	Short-term effects	Dangers
LSD (d-lysergic acid diethylamide)	Hallucinogen. Synthetic derivative of lysergic acid.	Swallowed, injected.	Euphoria, synesthesia, rapid mood shifts, depersonalization lasting 6-10 hours.	Recurrence of initial effects, panic or paranoid psychosis, hallucinations, delusions of grandeur, possible chromosome damage. Psychological dependence.
Marijuana (cannabis sativa)	Stimulant; mild hallucinogen. Made from the flower tops or leaves of the female hemp plant. Chief active ingredient: tetrahydrocannabinol.	Smoked, sniffed, swallowed.	Euphoria, mood swings, loss of inhibitions, distortion of time and space lasting 2-4 hours.	"Drop-out syndrome," possible panic or psychotic reactions. Psychological dependence.
Mescaline	Hallucinogen. Extract of peyote cactus.	Swallowed, injected, sniffed.	Exhilaration, anxiety, hallucinations lasting 6-12 hours.	Gastric distress, paranoid psychosis. Psychological dependence.
Morphine (morphine sulfate)	Depressant. Principal derivative of opium.	Swallowed, injected.	Euphoria, difficulty in concentrating lasting 4-8 hours.	Impaired breathing and intestinal activity, respiratory arrest. Psychological and physiological dependence.
Organic solvents (model glue, aerosols)	Stimulant. Chief active ingredient: toluene.	Sniffed.	Blurred vision, slurred speech, lack of coordination, hallucinations lasting 1-4 hours.	Nausea, vomiting, blood damage, paralysis of vocal cords, convulsions, respiratory arrest. Psychological dependence.
Psilocybin (phosphoryltryptamine)	Hallucinogen. Extract of Mexican mushroom.	Swallowed.	Nausea, vomiting, headaches lasting 6-8 hours.	Psychosis. Psychological dependence.
STP (dimethoxy-alphamethy-penylethylamine)	Hallucinogen. Derivative of amphetamine.	Swallowed.	Euphoria, confusion, hallucinations lasting 3-14 days.	Sudden violence, nerve impairment, psychosis, respiratory arrest, possible chromosome damage. Psychological dependence.

Reprinted from *Nursing Update*, Vol. 1, no. 3, 1970, p. 9, with permission from Miller and Fink Publishing Corporation, Darien, Conn.

First-Aid for Snake Venom Poisoning

Findlay E. Russell

Snake venom poisoning is an emergency requiring immediate attention and the exercise of considerable judgment. Delayed or inadequate treatment may result in tragic consequences. On the other hand, failure to differentiate between the bite of a venomous and a non-venomous snake may lead to the use of measures that can not only cause discomfort to the victim but may produce deleterious results. It is essential that a diagnosis be established before any treatment is instituted. In making the diagnosis it must be remembered that a venomous snake may bite a person without injecting venom, and that such bites are best treated as simple puncture wounds. It should also be borne in mind that some persons bitten by non-venomous snakes become excited and even hysterical, and that these emotions may give rise to disorientation, faintness, dizziness, rapid respiration or hyperventilation, a rapid pulse and even primary shock.

The person charged with the responsibility of instituting first-aid treatment will first need to determine whether or not envenomation has occurred. Secondly, he will need to decide, among other things, upon the kind of treatment to be used, and then how to initiate it with the greatest possible speed. Above all, he must *keep cool* and consider each move thoroughly. Any treatment, to be effective, must be instituted immediately following the bite and must include measures (1) to retard absorption of the venom; (2) to remove as much venom as possible from the wound; (3) to neutralize the venom; (4) to mitigate the effects produced by the venom; and (5) to prevent complications, including secondary infection.

Step One

Capture the Snake and Kill It

Make every effort to identify the snake before initiating treatment. If identification is not established at the time of the bite, make an effort to find the snake. Most snakes will remain in the immediate area of the accident and can be found quickly without too much difficulty. If a second person is present, send him in search of the snake while the victim remains at rest. Exercise extreme caution in hunting for the offending snake. A reptile that has bitten once is just as likely to bite again as not. The snake can be killed by a sharp blow on the head. *Do not* handle the snake. Carry it on a stick or in a cloth bag if it cannot be positively identified.

If the snake is a venomous one proceed with the first-aid measures as out-

Reprinted with permission from *Toxicon*, 1967, Vol. 4, pp. 285-289.

lined. Do not depend on the amount of pain or absence of pain as a symptom on which to base your decision on whether or not the offending snake was venomous.

Step Two

Apply a Constriction Band or Tourniquet

In cases of envenomation by most Crotalidae, a constriction band should be placed above the first joint proximal, or 2 to 4 in. proximal to the bite. It should be applied immediately following the bite and tight enough to occlude the superficial venous and lymphatic return but not the arterial flow. It should be released for 90 sec every 10 min. The constriction band can be moved in advance of the progressive swelling. It should be removed as soon as antivenin has been started or suction discontinued. In no case of viper venom poisoning should a constriction band be used for more than 2 hr. It is of little value if applied later than 30 min following the bite. It should be used in conjunction with incision and suction in viper bites.

In envenomation by elapids, the constriction band or tourniquet is of questionable value. However, in cases of severe envenomation by cobras, kraits, mambas, tiger snakes, death adders and taipans, a tight tourniquet should be applied immediately proximal to the bite and left in place until antivenin is given. It should be released for 90 sec every 10 min.

Step Three

Incision and suction

Incision and suction are of definite value when applied immediately following bites by the vipers, particularly the pit vipers of North America. They are of lesser value following bites by the South American vipers and Asiatic vipers, and probably of little value subsequent to envenomation by the elapids and sea snakes. This advice is based on clinical and experimental data which reflect upon the differences in the kind and depth of bites inflicted by the various venomous snakes, the rate and route of absorption of the venom, and the biochemical and physiopharmacological properties of the different snake venoms.

In viper bites, excluding those by small European vipers and small copperheads of North America, cruciate or longitudinal incisions of one-eighth to one-quarter in. in length should be made through the fang marks, except in those cases where there is an abnormal amount of bleeding or an obvious defect in coagulation. The incisions should be made as deep as the fang penetration, which in most rattlesnake bites is just through the skin. The direction of the animal's strike and the curvature of the fang should be borne in mind when determining the plane of incision. Suction should then be applied and continued for the first hour following the bite. Oral suction should not be used if other means of suction are available. Multiple incisions over the involved extremity or in advance of progressive edema are not advised. To be effective, suction must be applied within the first few minutes following the bite. It is of little value if delayed for 30 min or more. Incisions through the fang marks without subsequent suction are of questionable value and should be avoided.

In pit viper bites the proper application of the constriction band or tourniquet, and incision and suction have been found to be of definite value as first-aid measures (1-6). Their misapplication or late application have resulted in appraisals which do not always reflect a ready knowledge of the problem. In treating 104 rattlesnake bites over a period of 12 years, most of which arrived at the hospital following the initiation of some first-aid measures, the author has observed that those patients who properly applied a constriction band and incised the fang marks and applied suction fared better than seemingly similar cases where these measures were not used. In several patients we have been able to remove the exudate from the suction cups, and in a controlled experiment have demonstrated that the material was lethal to mice. In 30 cases of envenomation by elapids and African and Asian vipers we have observed that incision and suction were probably valueless as first-aid measures. These findings support the clinical observations of Reid (7) and Chapman (8).

Step Four

Immobilize the Injured Part

This can be done by splinting as for a broken leg. The immobilized part should then be kept below the level of the heart but not in a completely dependent position. If the wound is on the body, keep the victim in a sitting or lying position, depending on the location of the bite. The victim should always be kept warm. He should *not* be allowed to walk. He should *not* be given alcohol. He may be given water, coffee or tea. Any manifestations of fear or excitement should be alleviated by reassurance with encouraging words and actions.

Step Five

Transport the Patient to a Doctor or Hospital

This should be done by litter, if at all possible; if not, try to provide some other means of transportation. Do not let the victim walk if this can be avoided. Be sure to keep him warm, and the bitten part in a dependent position. If he must walk he should proceed slowly and rest periodically. Exertion must be avoided. If it appears that a period of more than one hour will pass before medical treatment can be given, the injured part should be kept cool with ice bags or cold cloths. This will produce some vasoconstriction and in some cases reduce pain. It has no effect on the chemistry of the deleterious fractions of the venom, nor should it be used in place of the constriction band and of incision and suction during the first hour following the bite.

Step Six

Antivenin

Under certain conditions antivenin may need to be given as a first-aid measure. Under no circumstances, however, should it be administered by an untrained person. Deaths have occurred following injection of antivenin in persons sensitive to horse serum (9). Antivenin might need to be given in those cases where severe symptoms and signs develop early in the course of the illness, or where a delay of 4 hr or more following viper venom poisoning or 2 hr or more following elapid venom poisoning is foreseen.

In such cases the antivenin should be given intramuscularly following appropriate skin or conjunctival tests. The antivenin should be given intramuscularly at a site distant from the wound. The antivenin should never be injected into a finger or toe, and it should be administered intravenously only by qualified personnel. As the amount of antivenin available will more than likely be limited, one unit (vial or package) will probably be all that can be administered. The earlier this is injected the better the results that can be expected. Remember, if the victim is in shock the antivenin will be absorbed slowly from an intramuscular site. In such cases the antivenin may need to be given intravenously, but only by a qualified person.

Step Seven

Disposition of Victim

At the doctor's office or hospital, inform the doctor of the genus of the snake involved (if known), or turn the dead, unidentified snake over to the doctor. Give approximate time between bite and arrival, and point out any constriction bands or tourniquets left in place. Give details on any antivenin or drugs given the patient. Report all unusual signs and symptoms.

Step Eight

Other Supportive Measures

Should any of the following sequelae to the bite develop while the victim is being taken to the doctor, consider these measures:

A. Shock. 1. Place patient in recumbent or shock position.
2. Maintain an adequate airway.
3. Keep patient comfortably warm.
4. Control any severe pain. This can usually be done with salicylates or codeine, if available.
5. Allay apprehension by reassuring words and actions.
6. Give oxygen.

B. Respiratory distress. 1. Clear airway.
2. Apply artificial respiration. As long as the patient's heart continues to beat he has a chance to recover, and this may occur even after many hours of artificial respiration. The push-pull methods are most effective in this type of poisoning. However, use any methods with which you are familiar. Mouth-to-mouth breathing with positive pressure to the chest in rhythm can be used. If a mechanical resuscitator is available, use it if you are qualifed.

C. Vomiting. Vomiting frequently occurs following certain types of snake venom poisoning. Precautions should be taken to see that the patient does not aspirate vomitus.

D. Excessive salivation. Place head in a position to permit adequate drainage of saliva. Keep airway clear.

E. Convulsions. No treatment should be given during the attack except that which will protect the patient from being injured (e.g., biting his tongue, etc.).

It is not a purpose of this paper to discuss or evaluate all of the first-aid treatments that have been suggested or advised for snake venom poisoning. Some 217 cures for snake venom poisoning have been described in the literature (9). Some of the more frequently suggested are: injecting potassium permanganate, ammonia, vinegar or oil into the wound, wrapping the liver of the offending snake or of a freshly-killed chicken over the wound, setting fire to the wound after applying gasoline, cryotherapy, eating various plants or raw meat, applying mud packs to the wound, soaking the injured part in excrement, washing the wound with plant juices, indulging in whiskey, taking antihistamatics, etc. These and the other so-called cures are more than historical curiosities. Whatever the source, they are hazardous: first, because they often involve dangerous methods; second, because they delay the use of effective therapeutic procedures. Snake venom poisoning is an accident highly variable in the gravity of its results. It is one in which the most fantastic remedy may gain its reputation among credulous people by having cured a malady that required no treatment whatever.

In conclusion it should be noted that there is no single therapeutic standard of procedure for all cases of snake venom poisoning. Rest, immobilization of the injured part and reassurance are indicated in every case, and in themselves are valuable therapeutic measures, but beyond these, few measures can be recommended for all cases of snakebite. Avoid using any first-aid measure that has not been evaluated; remember, most of the cures you will hear about have been evaluated and found to be useless.

Acknowledgements – The author is indebted to the Attending Staff Association of the Los Angeles County Hospital, and the National Institute of Allergy and Infectious Diseases (Grant AC 00273) for the support of studies upon which certain of the data have been drawn.

REFERENCES

1. Leopold, R.S. and Merriam, T.W., Jr. "The Effectiveness of Tourniquet, Incision and Suction in Snake Venom Removal." U.S. Navy. med. Field Res. Lab. Res. Proj. MR005.09-0020. 1.3:211, Nov. 1960.
2. Russell, F.E. and Emery, J.A. "Incision and Suction Following Injection of Rattlesnake Venom." *Am. J. med. Sci.* 241 (1961): 160.
3. Gennaro, J.F., Jr. "Observations on the Treatment of Snakebite in North America." In: *Venomous and Poisonous Animals and Noxious Plants of the Pacific Region.* Oxford: Pergamon Press, 1963, p. 427.
4. Seeley, S.F. (For, Ad Hoc Committee on Snakebite Therapy, National Research Council, National Academy of Sciences.) "Interim Statement on First-Aid Therapy for Bites by Venomous Snakes." *Toxicon* 1 (1963): 81.
5. Russell, F.E. "Snake Venom Poisoning." In: *Cyclopedia of Medicine, Surgery and the Specialities.* Volume II. Philadelphia: Davis, 1962, p. 197.
6. McCollough, N.C. and Gennaro, J.F., Jr. "Evaluation of Venomous Snake Bite in the Southern United States from Parallel Clinical and Laboratory Investigations." *J. Fla. Med. Ass.* 49 (1963): 959.
7. Reid, H.A. "Cobra-Bites." *Br. med. J.* 2 (1964): 540.
8. Chapman, D.S. "The Clinico-Pathology and Treatment of Snake Bite in South and Central Africa." Presented at the Symposium on Animal Venoms, São Paulo, Brazil, 19 July 1966.
9. Russell, F.E. and Scharffenberg, R.S. *Bibliography of Snake Venoms and Venomous Snakes.* West Covina, California: Bibliographic Associates, 1964.

First Aid and Treatment for Snakebite

Ray A. Petersen, M.H.Ed.

There have recently been some new innovations for treatment of poisonous pit viper snakebite. Dr. Clifford Snyder, chairman of the Division of Plastic Surgery at the University of Utah, is rated as one of the world's authorities on snakebite treatment. His research has shown that if the snakebite victim remains at rest, less than 20 percent of the venom will spread from the site of the bite within the first two hours. If this venom is removed the patient stands a very good chance of survival.

Several variables affect the potency of a bite. Children experience more envenomation than an adult because of less blood volume. The size, condition, and type of snake may alter the toxicity or volume of the venom. The site and effectiveness of the bite are important factors. Usually a bite will not enter a large blood vessel, but if this does occur the venom spreads rapidly and death usually occurs within a few minutes. Usually the venom travels slowly with the lymphatic system, especially if the person remains physically inactive. Another variable is the resistance of the victim. The healthier the victim the greater his resistance.

Dr. Snyder has some suggestions for assembling a snakebite kit. It should have a flat tourniquet (constriction band), two surgical prep sponges pre-saturated with alcohol and protected in foil, a disposable scalpel in sterile foil, and a kit of antivenin.

A snakebite is a deadly serious matter and Dr. Snyder recommends the following first aid procedures:
1. Keep the victim quiet. Rest extremity horizontally on a level with the heart. The victim should avoid excitement and exertion which may propel the venom into the general circulation more rapidly.
2. The snake should be killed and retrieved for positive identification if possible. Positive identification of the type of snake will enhance medical treatment. However, the first-aider should not exert himself to kill the snake. Often a bite has been inflicted by a nonpoisonous snake; first aid procedures are then the same as those followed for any superficial wound. More than one person has been given first aid and medical treatment for a poisonous snakebite when the snakebite was harmless.
3. Apply a flat tourniquet (constriction band) about three inches above the bite (between the bite and the heart) if the bite is on an arm or leg. It should be tight enough to stop venous blood flow and lymph flow but not arterial blood flow. The tourniquet should be loose enough so that a finger can be inserted beneath it without force. Once applied the tourniquet should be left in place. A released tourniquet speeds venom through the body.

4. Cleanse the bitten skin area with the alcohol sponges. With a sterile scalpel or knife make one straight incision that connects both fang marks. The incision should extend one-quarter inch past the fang marks. The incision should go no deeper than through the skin so that no underlying vessels, nerves or tendons are cut. Do not make cross incisions, for they heal poorly, cause scars, and are contradictory to basic surgery principles.

   A new medical approach to be used only by doctors is the excision of an ecliptical section of tissue one inch equidistant from the fang marks and to the depth of the muscle fascia. An excision within two hours will usually retrieve nearly eighty percent of the injected venom.

5. Squeeze venom gently from the incision with the fingers for thirty minutes or until a doctor takes over. Mechanical suction should be applied in a vigorous but not forceful manner. Bulb suction can retrieve about fifty percent of the venom in fifteen minutes; however, Dr. Snyder does not endorse the use of a suction cup because it can cause damage to the tissue. Mouth suction is not recommended because it can introduce oral bacteria.

6. If ice is available wrap it with a cloth and apply it gradually to the bite area. Do not bind it tightly to the skin. Leave it there for no longer than an hour. Be sure to move it away gradually. Sudden removal of ice will result in a sudden uptake of venom. Using ice for long periods of time can cause frostbite which could result in amputation.

7. Antivenin can be administered in the field in an emergency, but instructions contained in each package must be followed rigidly. The required skin test for allergy must have proven negative. Wyeth's intramuscular polyvalent antivenin is recommended. Antivenin counteracts or neutralizes the snake venom.

   A doctor and *only* a doctor can administer antivenin intra-arterially. It then reaches the venom quicker than intravenous, intramuscular, or direct injections surrounding the wound. It is put in the brachial artery for upper extremities and in the femoral artery for lower extremities, and in the common carotid for head and neck bites.

8. Get the victim to a doctor or hospital as quickly as possible, but without exertion on his part. The victim should be under a doctor's observation for at least twenty-four hours following the bite.

   Every year in this country about 1500 snakebites occur, of which about 45 result in death. If proper first aid procedures are immediately carried out, followed by proper medical treatment, victims have a high chance of survival.

   Dr. Snyder feels that many first aid manuals give outdated and improper instructions on caring for snakebite. Many people have suffered needless pain and permanent disfigurement from improper first aid and medical treatment. He is engaged in a campaign to remedy this situation.

Man versus Arthropods

Cyril H. March, M.D. and Alexander A. Fisher, M.D.

Arthropods (insects and arachnids) affect man by provoking toxic, allergic or mixed reactions. The local and systemic toxic reaction is exemplified by the bite of the brown recluse spider. Large doses of cortiocosteroids are helpful in many of these syndromes. Intralesional steroids can be beneficial in papular urticaria produced by fleas and bedbugs. Eradication of caterpillar dermatitis requires washing of the clothing and bedding contaminated by the venomous caterpillar hair. At present, topical repellents offer the best protection.

Direct contact of man with arthropods may result in a wide variety of reactions, most of which are limited to the skin. The arthropods of dermatologic interest include arachnids (spiders, ticks and mites) and insects (lice, flies, fleas, beetles, caterpillars, bees and wasps). *Table 1* lists the differences between these classes.

TABLE 1. DIFFERENCES BETWEEN ARACHNIDS AND INSECTS

Characteristics	Arachnids	Insects
Number of legs	Eight	Six
Thorax, head and abdomen	Fused	Separate
Wings	None	Present in most species
Antennae	None	Single pair

The biophysiologic mechanisms by which arthropods affect man and by which man reacts to contact with the arachnid or insect fall into three categories: (1) *toxic,* in which the major damage is inflicted by poisons or venoms injected by the pest; (2) *allergic,* in which the major damage is due to the reaction of the host to normally nontoxic substances, and (3) *mixed,* in which both toxic and allergic mechanisms are operative.

Other damaging effects, which will not be discussed here, include: the role of arthropods as vectors of disease; secondary infections following excoriations, poor hygiene or direct introduction of bacteria by parasites, and delusions of parasitosis, an often puzzling, fascinating and recalcitrant disorder. Space limitations also preclude the description of some parasites which have had great impor-

Reprinted with permission from *Family Physician*, October 1967, pp. 52-56.

tance in the past, such as *Sarcoptes scabiei* (variety hominis), the itch mite of scabies, and *Pediculus humanus* (variety corporis), the body louse harbored in clothing. Because of the relative rarity of human scabies, the physician may not recognize the occasional case he may encounter, especially in patients with good personal hygiene and relatively minor lesions. Animal scabies (particularly the canine variety) may also cause dermatitis in man. Although pediculosis corporis is now rare, cases of pediculosis pubic (due to *Phthirius pubis*) are encountered fairly regularly. This is probably attributable to the increase in sexual promiscuity in the age group between 15 and 30.

Toxic Reactions

The brown recluse spider (*Loxosceles reclusus*) introduces a potent poison through its bite. The resulting skin reaction is called "necrotic arachnidism." Systemic reactions also occur and are sometimes fatal.

The spider is of particular interest to inhabitants of south central United States. It is found inside old houses, in cracks in walls, behind pictures or furniture and inside clothing. It does not attack unless molested. The local reaction to its bite is delayed for several hours and is manifested by local pain, ischemia and ecchymosis, followed by the formation of a bleb. Several days later, when the initial local reaction appears to have subsided, dry gangrene develops in the skin, with eschar formation and deep ulceration which may require extensive grafting.

The systemic reaction following the bite develops within a few hours and consists of fever, chills, malaise, nausea, vomiting and joint pains. A generalized morbilliform rash as well as purpura may be present. The latter is due to thrombocytopenia which is accompanied by leukocytosis and sometimes by hemolytic anemia (hemoglobinemia, hemoglobinuria and jaundice). The systemic manifestations subside within one week. The best treatment currently available is the administration of antihistamines and large doses of corticosteroids. A specific antiserum has been devised for necrotic arachnidism following the bite of a South American spider closely related to the brown recluse spider.

Blister Beetle Dermatitis

Numerous varieties of blister beetles are found in the United States, primarily in the southeastern or western states. Agricultural workers are often exposed since the beetles feed on various flowering plants, potatoes, clover and soybeans.

Blister beetles are 1/2 to 1 inch long, soft, long-legged and very agile. In the United States they mature in the summer and disappear in the winter, which accounts for a strictly seasonal incidence. These insects contain the toxic agent cantharidin. Little or no cantharidin is excreted if the beetle is allowed to walk undisturbed across the skin but the slightest pressure on its body causes a clear amber fluid to exude from the knee joints, prothorax and genitalia. Mild tingling of the skin may develop in about 10 minutes, followed in eight to 12 hours by a flaccid bulla without surrounding inflamation. A good-sized bulla may develop if the insect is crushed on the skin. Often the victim unknowingly brushes off the insect and is later surprised to find blisters which seem to have come from nowhere. Blister beetles are strongly attracted to light and contact the skin mostly at night, so that patients discover the blisters in the morning. The blisters occur on exposed parts, frequently in a linear arrangement.

Treatment of the blisters consists of careful removal of the beetle *without crushing*, washing the area with solvents, such as acetone and benzene, and then cleansing with soap and water to remove the vesicant material (cantharidin). Further local treatment is the same as for burns.

Allergic Reactions

The material injected into the skin by bite or sting may or may not be toxic. If it is toxic, the initial reaction causes temporary discomfort. However, because of the antigenicity of the material, repeated biting or stinging causes a severe reaction (anaphylactic shock) or a prolonged local reaction, such as papular urticaria.

Bee, Yellow Jacket and Wasp Stings

These insects are common throughout the United States. Local reaction following the sting is due to the release of toxic substances which cause inflammation, swelling and pain. This reaction can generally be controlled by the application of ice to the sting area and the use of oral antihistamines.

After single or repeated stinging, antibodies develop in the sensitized individual and a new sting will produce an allergic reaction which may vary from prolonged local inflammation to urticaria, angioneurotic edema, malaise, weakness, collapse and even death from anaphylactic shock. When moderate, these manifestations may be controlled by orally administered antihistamines and/or steroids. However, if the reaction is severe, the patient may require epinephrine (1:1000) intramuscularly as well as oxygen inhalation and plasma intravenously.

Patients known to be sensitive to wasp and bee stings should carry epinephrine whenever there is a risk of exposure. Desensitization through repeated injections of small, graduated doses of prepared antigens must be considered for highly sensitive patients. This can be accomplished through a course of immunization with commercially prepared antigen from crushed insects (Hollister-Stier) or with the pure venom of the incriminated insect, followed by yearly revaccination (Loveless). Although the latter procedure is preferable, it requires highly specialized facilities for the collection of pure venom and is available only in a few large centers. Desensitization with commercial antigen, although somewhat less satisfactory, gives a fair amount of protection and is available everywhere.

Papular Urticaria from Fleas, Bedbugs and Mosquitoes

Papular urticaria is also known as lichen urticatus, prurigo simplex and strophulus pruriginosus. There is more cellular inflammation exudate in the lesions of papular urticaria than in simple hives. This exudate causes the lesions to persist for several days, weeks or even months, in contrast to the fleeting character of ordinary urticaria. Occasionally, classic urticaria and even angiodema may accompany urticaria of the papular variety.

The reaction seems to occur more often among children with an atopic background and, in certain types of skin, any insect bite may cause a prolonged local reaction similar to a very small area of lichen simplex (localized neuro-dermatitis). The insects most commonly responsible for papular urticaria are the following:

1. The flea (*Pulex irritans*). These insects are common throughout the United States, although they are more prevalent in areas with poor hygiene. (A particular type is found on the West Coast, especially in San Francisco and San Diego.) After several months or years of exposure to flea bites, the papular urticaria type of allergic response eventually wanes and is replaced by a normal, transient reaction.

2. The bedbug (*Cimex lectularius*). These insects are encountered primarily in areas of poor hygiene. Bedbugs remain on the clothing or bed linen from which they emerge to feed at night. They are active migrants and pass readily from one person to another. Since bedbugs can withstand long periods of starvation, even uninhabited areas may continue to be infested.

3. The mosquito (*Culicidae*). These insects are widespread in all areas in which there is stagnant water. Mosquito bites cause much discomfort because of the severe pruritus which accompanies the early reaction in certain individuals. This reaction may persist for weeks or months.

Control of Papular Urticaria Due to Insects

Several simple measures help eliminate insects which cause papular urticaria. A spray of 5 percent DDT* should be used daily in the house. The baseboards, cellar, bed frames and upholstered furniture should receive special attention. A powder of 5 percent DDT should be dusted under cushions and rugs and wherever the spray cannot be used. All collections of sand around the house must be removed since they can harbor live flea eggs for as long as a year.

*Editors' Note: Since the use of DDT is prohibited in many areas the use of a suitable substitute is recommended.

Contact with dogs and cats should be avoided if possible. Pet dogs should be dusted with 5 percent DDT powder once weekly for three weeks. Since cats may become sick from licking DDT, they should be dusted with pyrethrum flea powder. Sleeping quarters for pets should be provided with padding which can easily be removed, cleaned and aired.

Until the infestation is under control, insect repellent may be applied to the exposed skin of the patient.

Treatment of Papular Urticaria

The treatment of papular urticaria requires elimination of the cause as outlined previously. Topical measures include the use of antipruritic lotions and steroids, which decrease the itch and prevent the self-perpetuation of lesions. Oral antihistamines are sometimes helpful. However, the treatment of choice is intralesional infiltration of triamcinolone acetonide or similar steroid. A small amount (0.1 to 0.3 cc.) of 5 or 10 mg. per cc. suspension is infiltrated into each papule, deep in the dermis or in the subdermal tissue. Relief is obtained within a few hours and the lesions involute within eight to 10 days.

Mixed Reactions

Caterpillar Dermatitis

Caterpillar dermatitis may occur anywhere in the United States. Epidemics of caterpillar dermatitis (urticaria epidemica) are occasionally seen in Texas during the migration of caterpillars. Several varieties can produce skin reactions, particularly the puss caterpillar (*Megalopyge opercularis*) and the brown-tail moth (*Euproctis phaeorrhoea*). These caterpillars and moths possess venomous bristly hair or spines (*setae*) which can pierce the skin on contact and cause nonallergic urticarial eruption. The lesions may persist for several days. Occasionally the dermatitis may simulate an allergic contact reaction such as poison ivy dermatitis.

Clothing and bedding which may have become contaminated with hair must be washed. The local reaction is best treated with cold, wet compresses and corticosteroid creams. In rare cases, widespread exposure may cause systemic reactions which require the administration of epinephrine and cortiocosteroids.

Chigger Bites

Chiggers (*Trombicula irritans*) are found throughout the United States but are definitely more prevalent in the South. The tiny red larvae of these mites bury themselves into unprotected areas of the victim's skin and suck tissue fluids. Hunters, campers and farmers often complain of this type of bite. The reaction to the bite may be solely pruritic or it may be complicated by eczematous reactions, even after the larva has dropped off. In some instances, a persistent papule with an ulcerated center will develop.

Chigger bites can be prevented by wearing proper clothing and boots. Treatment consists of local antipruritic agents, corticosteroid creams and intralesional corticosteroids as described in the treatment of urticaria. An ice cube pressed on the lesion often gives considerable relief. The application of clear nail lacquer is a popular remedy for relief of the itch from chigger bites. Rarely, persistent lesions may require cryotherapy, electrodesiccation or even surgical removal. Histologically as well as clinically, the papule or nodule may mimic the appearance of such neoplasms as lymphomas or sarcomas. For this reason, persistent reactions which may have followed insect bites must be evaluated with extreme care.

Protection Against Arthropods

Mass eradication of pests is an important public health problem. Every year, large sums of money are spent in government programs for this purpose as well as for the development of new control methods. These new approaches involve the use of chemosterilants (substances which prevent reproduction) and radiosterilants and the release of sterile male insects to curb reproduction of the species.

Protection of the individual is of greater interest to the physician. Considerable research is being devoted to substances which repel or block the attraction of insects to man. Some of these substances are present on the skin surface, probably in the lipid fraction. Also, certain sweat constituents appear to attract some insects. The possibility of developing repellents which are active when taken orally is also being investigated. This would represent a great advance in protection against arthropods.

The only practical agents at present are those which block the impulse to probe — the topical repellents. They are convenient, effective against several species of annoying arthropods and unlikely to have systemic effects. Some of the disadvantages of topical repellents are that they wear off quickly, they might not cover all exposed skin areas and they might irritate the skin. Other inconveniences are their odor, their oiliness and their softening effect on paint, lacquer and synthetic fabrics.

At present, the best all-purpose repellent, particularly against mosquitoes, is DET (diethyltoluamide). It also repels ticks, chiggers, fleas and leeches. DET is contained in numerous commercial preparations, which are available either as sprays or as liquids. One recent preparation combines the repellent with a sunscreen agent.

Other effective repellents are dimethyl carbamate, dimethyl phthalate (good for mosquitoes and chiggers), ethohexadiol and benzyl benzoate. A good chigger repellent is 5 percent precipitated sulfur in a vanishing-cream base.

Impregnation of clothing is an effective method of protection against insect or chigger bites. This measure is used whenever there is heavy exposure and is especially suitable for forest rangers, hunters, fishermen and campers. The repellent should be applied to both the clothes and the skin. DET, diluted to 5 percent strength in water, may be sprayed or brushed on clothing. However, DET is removed by washing whereas benzyl benzoate will remain.

Because of the speed of air travel, some unlikely dermatologic eruptions due to insects appear in unexpected geographic locations. Recently, cases of "ver du cayor" (an equatorial African form of myiasis) have been reported in Manhattan and Wisconsin and a case of tungiasis has been seen in New York City.

Bugs and Bites

The giant tarantula crushed cars and knocked over buildings as it moved steadily onward toward the high school gymnasium, where the residents of the little Arizona town cowered in fear, praying that the Army would get there in time with the lethal freezing spray.

Unfortunately, science fiction films with scenes like the one described have given a bad name to one of North America's most helpful bugs, the tarantula.

Believe it or not, the huge, hairy, eight-legged creature found in the Southwestern United States usually will not bite unless teased into it, and then the bite is no more harmful than a pinprick.

Tarantulas found in tropical areas have a more venomous bite that can cause local pain and swelling, but the spiders are still not considered deadly. As a matter of fact, the tarantulas that inhabit the United States are beneficial because they destroy harmful insects.

If you see a tarantula, leave it alone. If you should be bitten by one, wash the bite and apply antiseptic to prevent infection.

The tarantula has a bad reputation by mistake, but there are several other kinds of bugs that have earned bad names.

Bees, for example, kill more people in this country than any other venomous creature. A 10-year study of 460 deaths from bites or stings shows that the insect group *Hymenoptera* (bees, wasps, hornets, ants) caused 50 percent of these fatalities. Snakes caused 30 percent, spiders 14 percent, and scorpions 2 percent of the deaths.

In many persons a bee sting causes only a painful swelling that will go away in a few hours. But in other persons the insect venom causes an allergic reaction that can vary from dizziness to headaches, from abdominal cramps to extreme nausea, from itching to death.

Fortunately, the first allergic reaction to an insect bite will not be fatal and can provide a warning to the victim.

If you notice any of the warning signs named or experience difficulty breathing, or have hives and swelling in a spot different from the location of the sting, see a doctor right away. You can be treated for the reaction and also may be immunized against future reactions.

Once a person is sensitized to the venom of one kind of *Hymenoptera*, he will be allergic to the sting of them all.

There are some things you can do to avoid being stung. Sweet smells attract

Reprinted with permission from *School Safety*, March/April 1971, Vol. 6, No. 4, pp. 15-18.

	DESCRIPTION	HABITAT	PROBLEM
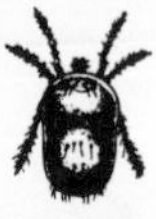 **CHIGGER**	Oval with red velvety covering. Sometimes almost colorless. Larva has six legs. Harmless adult has eight and resembles a small spider. Very tiny— about 1/20-inch long.	Found in low damp places covered with vegetation: shaded woods, high grass or weeds, fruit orchards. Also lawns and golf courses. From Canada to Argentina.	Attaches itself to the skin by inserting mouthparts into a hair follicle. Injects a digestive fluid that causes cells to disintegrate. Then feeds on cell parts. It does not suck blood.
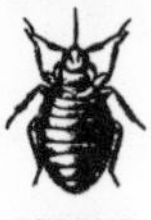 **BEDBUG**	Flat oval body with short broad head and six legs. Adult is reddish brown. Young are yellowish white. Unpleasant pungent odor. From ⅛ to ¼-inch in length.	Hides in crevices, mattresses, under loose wallpaper during day. At night travels considerable distance to find victims. Widely distributed throughout the world.	Punctures the skin wtih piercing organs and sucks blood. Local inflammation and welts result from anticoagulant enzyme that bug secretes from salivary glands while feeding.
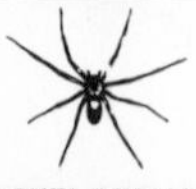 **BROWN RECLUSE SPIDER**	Oval body with eight legs. Light yellow to medium dark brown. Has distinctive mark shaped like a fiddle on its back. Body from ⅜ to ½-inch long, ¼-inch wide, ¾-inch from toe-to-toe.	Prefers dark places where it's seldom disturbed. Outdoors: old trash piles, debris and rough ground. Indoors: attics, storerooms, closets. Found in Southern and Midwestern U.S.	Bites producing an almost painless sting that may not be noticed at first. Shy, it bites only when annoyed or surprised. Left alone, it won't bite. Victim rarely sees the spider.
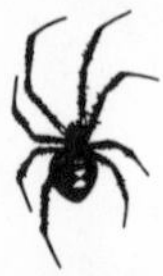 **BLACK WIDOW SPIDER**	Color varies from dark brown to glossy black. Densely covered with short microscopic hairs. Red or yellow hourglass marking on the underside of the female's abdomen. Male does not have this mark and is not poisonous. Overall length with legs extended is 1½ inch. Body is ¼-inch wide.	Found with eggs and web. Outside: in vacant rodent holes, under stones, logs, in long grass, hollow stumps and brush piles. Inside: in dark corners of barns, garages, piles of stone, wood. Most bites occur in outhouses. Found in Southern Canada, throughout U.S., except Alaska.	Bites causing local redness. Two tiny red spots may appear. Pain follows almost immediately. Larger muscles become rigid. Body temperature rises slightly. Profuse perspiration and tendency toward nausea follow. It's usually difficult to breathe or talk. May cause constipation, urine retention.
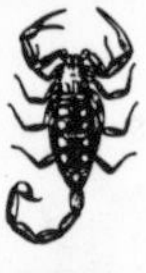 **SCORPION**	Crablike appearance with clawlike pincers. Fleshy postabdomen or "tail" has 5 segments, ending in a bulbous sac and stinger. Two poisonous types: solid straw yellow or yellow with irregular black stripes on back. From 2½ to 4 inches.	Spends days under loose stones, bark, boards, floors of outhouses. Burrows in the sand. Roams freely at night. Crawls under doors into homes. Lethal types are found only in the warm desert-like climate of Arizona and adjacent areas.	Stings by thrusting its tail forward over its head. Swelling or discoloration of the area indicates a non-dangerous, though painful, sting. A dangerously toxic sting doesn't change the appearance of the area, which does become hypersensitive.
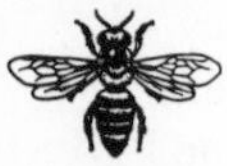 **BEE**	Winged body with yellow and black stripes. Covered with branched or feathery hairs. Makes a buzzing sound. Different species vary from ½ to 1 inch in length.	Lives in aerial or underground nests or hives. Widely distributed throughout the world wherever there are flowering plants—from the polar regions to the equator.	Stings with tail when annoyed. Burning and itching with localized swelling occur. Usually leaves venom sac in victim. It takes between 2 and 3 minutes to inject all the venom.
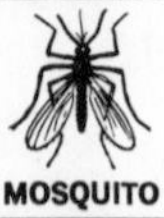 **MOSQUITO**	Small dark fragile body with transparent wings and elongated mouthparts. From ⅛ to ¼-inch long.	Found in temperate climates throughout the world where the water necessary for breeding is available.	Bites and sucks blood. Itching and localized swelling result. Bite may turn red. Only the female is equipped to bite.
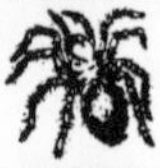 **TARANTULA**	Large dark "spider" with a furry covering. From 6 to 7 inches in toe-to-toe diameter.	Found in Southwestern U.S. and the tropics. Only the tropical varieties are poisonous.	Bites produce pin-prick sensation with negligible effect. It will not bite unless teased.
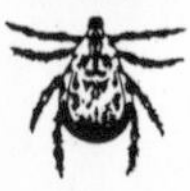 **TICK**	Oval with small head; the body is not divided into definite segments. Grey or brown. Measures from ¼-inch to ¾-inch when mature.	Found in all U.S. areas and in parts of Southern Canada, on low shrubs, grass and trees. Carried around by both wild and domestic animals.	Attaches itself to the skin and sucks blood. After removal there is danger of infection, especially if the mouthparts are left in the wound.

SEVERITY	TREATMENT	PROTECTION	
Itching from secreted enzymes results several hours after contact. Small red welts appear. Secondary infection often follows. Degree of irritation varies with individuals.	Lather with soap and rinse several times to remove chiggers. If welts have formed, dab antiseptic on area. Severe lesions may require antihistamine ointment.	Apply proper repellent to clothing, particularly near uncovered areas such as wrists and ankles. Apply to skin. Spray or dust infested areas (lawns, plants)with suitable chemicals.	**CHIGGER**
Affects people differently. Some have marked swelling and considerable irritation while others aren't bothered. Sometimes transmits serious diseases.	Apply antiseptic to prevent possible infection. Bug usually bites sleeping victim, gorges itself completely in 3-5 minutes and departs. It's rarely necessary to remove one.	Spray beds, mattresses, bed springs and baseboards with insecticide. Bugs live in large groups. They migrate to new homes on water pipes and clothing.	**BEDBUG**
In two to eight hours pain may be noticed followed by blisters, swelling, hemorrhage or ulceration. Some people experience rash, nausea, jaundice, chills, fever, cramps or joint pain.	Summon doctor. Bite may require hospitalization for a few days. Full healing may take from 6-8 weeks. Weak adults and children have been known to die.	Use caution when cleaning secluded areas in the home or using machinery usually left idle. Check firewood, inside shoes, packed clothing and bedrolls — frequent hideaways.	**BROWN RECLUSE SPIDER**
Venom is more dangerous than a rattlesnake's but is given in much smaller amounts. About 5 per cent of bite cases result in death. Death is from asphyxiation due to respiratory paralysis. More dangerous for children, to adults its worst feature is pain. Convulsions result in some cases.	Use an antiseptic such as alcohol or hydrogen peroxide on the bitten area to prevent secondary infection. Keep victim quiet and call a doctor. Do not treat as you would a snakebite since this will only increase the pain and chance of infection; bleeding will not remove the venom.	Wear gloves when working in areas where there might be spiders. Destroy any egg sacs you find. Spray insecticide in any area where spiders are usually found, especially under privy seats. Check them out regularly. General cleanliness, paint and light discourage spiders.	**BLACK WIDOW SPIDER**
Excessive salivation and facial contortions may follow. Temperature rises to over 104°. Tongue becomes sluggish. Convulsions, in waves of increasing intensity, may lead to death from nervous exhaustion. First 3 hours most critical.	Apply tourniquet. Keep victim quiet and call a doctor immediately. Do not cut the skin or give pain killers. They increase the killing power of the venom. Antitoxin, readily available to doctors, has proved to be very effective.	Apply a petroleum distillate to any dwelling places that cannot be destroyed. Cats are considered effective predators as are ducks and chickens, though the latter are more likely to be stung and killed. Don't go barefoot at night.	**SCORPION**
If a person is allergic, more serious reactions occur—nausea, shock, unconsciousness. Swelling may occur in another part of the body. Death may result.	Gently scrape (don't pluck) the stinger so venom sac won't be squeezed. Wash with soap and antiseptic. If swelling occurs, contact doctor. Keep victim warm while resting.	Have exterminator destroy nests and hives. Avoid wearing sweet fragrances and bright clothing. Keep food covered. Move slowly or stand still in the vicinity of bees.	**BEE**
Sometimes transmits yellow fever, malaria, encephalitis and other diseases. Scratching can cause secondary infections.	Don't scratch. Lather with soap and rinse to avoid infection. Apply antiseptic to relieve itching.	Destroy available breeding water to check multiplication. Place nets on windows and beds. Use proper repellent.	**MOSQUITO**
Usually no more dangerous than a pin prick. Has only local effects.	Wash and apply antiseptic to prevent the possibility of secondary infection.	Harmless to man, the tarantula is beneficial since it destroys harmful insects.	**TARANTULA**
Sometimes carries and spreads Rocky Mountain spotted fever, tularemia, Colorado tick fever. In a few rare cases, causes paralysis until removed.	Apply heated needle to tick. Gently remove with tweezers so none of the mouthparts are left in skin. Wash with soap and water; apply antiseptic.	Cover exposed parts of body when in tick-infested areas. Use proper repellent. Remove ticks attached to clothes, body. Check neck and hair. Bathe.	**TICK**

bees, so avoid strong perfumes and hair sprays, hair tonics and sun tan lotion. Floral fragrances in particular seem attractive.

Brightly colored clothing or flowery prints and black or dark colors seem to anger insects, according to some experts, so wear dull white, dark green or khaki for outdoor activities, and always wear shoes.

Uncovered food attracts bees as well as other insects. Keep food covered if possible and don't leave garbage in uncovered containers.

When a bee is around, avoid swift movements. If a bee lands on you, by all means, don't slap at it as you would a fly or mosquito. A bee won't sting unless threatened.

More adults than children have fatal reactions to *Hymenoptera* stings. This may be due to the fact that allergic reactions to insect stings are cumulative — the first sting sensitizes the victim and more stings cause increasingly severe reactions. It is important to recognize the first sign of an allergic reaction to avoid future trouble.

The stings or bites of other creepy crawlers are more fatal to children than adults. Even a small amount of the venom of a scorpion or brown recluse spider may have an immediate and deadly effect on a small child.

Reactions to bites vary with individuals, too. Some people don't feel chigger bites, while others get watery lesions and even fever from them. Most people are not bothered by a bedbug bite, but it may be very irritating to others.

Sometimes the danger is not from the bite itself but from the secondary infection that may develop if the bite is not properly treated. Mosquito, bedbug and tick bites aren't very painful, but they can spread serious diseases, and infection from scratching or other contamination can be troublesome.

A tick can also produce a rare condition — paralysis leading to death. A healthy 4-year-old girl in Tennessee awoke one morning unable to make her arms and legs move correctly. While administering neurological tests at the hospital, doctors discovered a common wood tick on her head. Two hours after it was removed, she was able to walk across the room. She quickly returned to normal. Mysteriously, removal of the tick cured the paralysis.

Scorpions can be extremely dangerous. The venom of two species of scorpions found in Arizona and adjacent areas is lethal. It attacks the nervous system, causing convulsions that can lead to death. The victim is easily misled about the seriousness of the sting because it does not produce swelling or discoloration, although the area will become abnormally sensitive.

With the exception of these two Southwest species, the venom of most scorpions causes the flesh to swell and discolor. A 60-year-old man in Miami, Florida, was stung by a scorpion that he tried to pick up with only a facial tissue in his hand. His arm became swollen and paralyzed. He said later it was the most painful thing that had ever happened to him. Although frightening and uncomfortable, this kind of sting is not fatal.

Scorpion sting victims should be kept as quiet as possible and medical help sought immediately.

Never take pain-killing drugs if you are bitten by any poisonous creature — they increase the venom's lethal power.

Of course, your best protection is to avoid being bitten. Know your "bugs" — what they look like, where to find them, and how to avoid them. The chart on pages 124 and 125 will help you.

How (and How Not) to Treat Poison Ivy

Each year, some two million Americans suffer from poison-ivy dermatitis, one of the most common allergic disorders. It results from contact with the sap of such plants as poison ivy, poison oak and poison sumac. The incidence of poison-ivy dermatitis reaches its peak in the spring and early summer, when sap flows freely and leaves are tender and easily bruised. While direct contact with plants is the most common cause of poison-ivy dermatitis, the sensitizing material may reach the skin indirectly, by way of contaminated shoes and clothing, the fur of dogs and cats, golf-club heads, and even smoke from a bonfire in which poison ivy is burned along with debris. So potent is the allergen that it has been known to trigger allergic reactions in highly sensitive persons when present on the skin in such minute quantities as less than one part per million. And the allergen is durable: Traces of it on contaminated clothing can remain active for a year or longer.

Resistance to poison-ivy allergy varies widely from one individual to the next, and also at different periods of an individual's life. Adults are less likely than children to contact the dermatitis, because natural resistance to the allergen tends to increase with age. But according to the U.S. Public Health Service, at least seven persons out of ten are potentially allergic to the toxic sap; and they may be unexpectedly sensitized to it in middle age or later. So even after long years of apparent "natural immunity," it's prudent to behave as though you had become susceptible to poison-ivy dermatitis overnight.

Poison ivy, poison oak and poison sumac all cause substantially the same symptoms and require substantially the same treatment. The dermatitis usually starts with a rash that appears 24 to 48 hours after the sap has come in contact with the skin (although that period may be as short as a few hours or as long as a week). The skin reddens and itches or burns to a degree that may range from mild to intense, depending on the individual's susceptibility and the severity of exposure. Affected skin may weep a clear fluid, and, in more serious cases, swell and develop large blisters filled with that fluid. Popular opinion to the contrary, the fluid itself does not spread the dermatitis if the blisters are broken, as they might be in scratching. But scratching may in fact spread the dermatitis if minute quantities of the sap lodge under the nails; scratching may also lead to secondary infections, such as abscesses, if the skin is broken.

Reprinted with permission from *Consumer Reports*, June 1970, Vol. 35, No. 6, pp. 372-374. Copyright 1970 by Consumers Union of United States, Inc., a nonprofit organization.

Persistent or severe poison-ivy dermatitis can be dangerous as well as painful. If it affects genital, anal or facial areas extensively, the disorder should be treated by a physician. With severe involvement of the face, for example, the eyelids may swell shut. In serious cases such complications as fever, swollen lymph nodes, flu-like symptoms, kidney damage and even blood changes are possible. And in extreme cases, hospitalization may be necessary. (Where dermatitis is persistent, consider the possibility of repeated contamination by sap deposited, for example, on clothing. Thorough washing or dry-cleaning will effectively decontaminate such clothing.)

The Quest for Prevention

Americans are currently spending about $20 million a year on over-the-counter products sold for the prevention or relief of poison-ivy dermatitis. A recent issue of the "Pink Book," published for the drug trade, listed 66 such products; but their value is open to question. Preventive agents, whose purpose is to keep the poison from acting on the skin, fall into three main groups:

Washing Agents and Solvents

Strong laundry soap has long been used as a poison-ivy preventive, despite its limited effectiveness. The soap's lather, when allowed to dry on the skin, has reportedly given good protection to some highly sensitized persons; left overlong on the skin, however, the lather itself may act as an irritant and cause unwelcome reactions. Washing after exposure to the sap, a procedure commonly recommended, is often impractical or impossible when you're outdoors. And when washing is possible, it may be ineffective because of the speed with which the allergen acts on the skin. *The Medical Letter*, a nonprofit publication on drugs and therapeutics, considers that soap-and-water washing *may* be helpful if done within a few minutes of contact; washing as much as an hour after contact, according to another source, might benefit mildly sensitive persons. But not even prompt washing followed with applications of rubbing alcohol can protect some highly sensitive individuals from severe dermatitis. Other soaps (tincture of green soap, for example) and solvents such as acetone are unlikely to provide better protection.

Barrier Creams and Ointments

Creams and ointments meant to keep the allergen off the skin have been judged generally unsatisfactory. Clinically tested, such "barrier" ingredients as perborate, ferric chloride and white petroleum were only occasionally effective in shutting out the allergen. After a series of careful tests, Dr. Albert M. Kligman, a leading authority on poison-ivy dermatitis, dismissed the silicone creams, widely promoted about a decade ago, as "valueless." And in a study published by the American Medical Association in its *Archives of Dermatology*, Dr. Kligman wrote that "barrier creams offer no practical degree of protection against poison ivy dermatitis."

Detoxicants

Poison-ivy dermatitis might be preventable if the chemical irritant in the allergen could be neutralized by other chemicals. Some of the chemicals tested as detoxicants have in fact neutralized the poison under laboratory conditions; but none, so far, has proven clinically effective, presumably because their action is too slow to keep fast-acting allergen from penetrating the skin. Over a two-year period, Dr. Kligman tested more than 30 chemicals that might be expected to abort dermatitis, applying them, in general, an hour before exposure and an hour after it. None had any significant clinical effect.

One of the ineffective chemicals Dr. Kligman tested was zirconium, for which enthusiastic – and groundless – claims have been made. Some over-the-counter products used in the treatment of dermatitis contain zirconium, usually in the form of salts or hydrous zirconium oxide. Of 17 brands mentioned in the "Handbook of Non-Prescription Drugs," eight are noted to contain zirconium: *Allergesic, Antivy, Calamatum Skin Relief, Histonium, RhuliCream, RhuliSpray, Ziradryl* and *Zotox*. The zirconium is usually in small amounts – from 1 to 4 percent – but *Zotox* ointment is claimed to contain 21 percent zirconia, the equivalent of about 16 percent zirconium. (Other sources mention zirconium in *Calamatum Aerosol Spray, Ivy-Eze, Rhucen* and some over-the-counter products apparently no longer manufactured.) In whatever amounts, however, "controlled clinical experience . . . has shown . . . (zirconium) to be valueless" as a preventive, according to an article in *The Journal of the American Medical Association* for December 7, 1964.

But besides being ineffective, zirconium may be downright harmful. Even in minute quantities, it may cause granulomas – small, hard, painless lumps in the skin – in susceptible persons. The granulomas, which can be unsightly, usually last for periods ranging from several months to many years. Moreover, some zirconium-sensitive individuals might not realize the granulomas had been caused by a poison-ivy remedy, since the lumps may not appear until as much as eight to ten weeks after contact with the chemical. In CU's view, zirconium should be banished from all products sold for the treatment of poison ivy as it has been – and for the same reason – from almost all antiperspirant products.

Some physicians believe that extracts of the poison-ivy plant, injected or administered orally, can hyposensitize – build up immunity to the dermatitis. While that preventive treatment has been effective with some individuals, its drawbacks are numerous. Hyposensitization is at best temporary, expensive and relatively inconvenient; the extracts must be administered gradually over a period of many months; and in highly sensitive persons, "complete sensitization . . . is not possible with any dosage" of the injectable type, according to Dr. Kligman. "All that can be expected is a reduction in sensitivity (briefer or less generalized, less intense attacks)." Dosages containing active allergen must be conservative, too, and carefully graded to avoid a variety of adverse side effects, some of which may be severe. (The danger of such effects is somewhat lower with oral dosages than with injections.) So hyposensitizing is probably indicated only for severely allergic persons who cannot avoid contact with the allergen.

Treatments

Remedies held beneficial in treating the dermatitis have ranged over the years "from the preposterous to the fantastic," in Dr. Kligman's phrase: coffee, cream, buttermilk, kerosene, iodine, marshmallow, mustard and gunpowder, among others, and a variety of botanical preparations. Physicians have endorsed certain remedies, too, without conclusive testing of them, because of their apparent effectiveness with certain patients (despite the wide diversity of individual reactions to the allergy). But most cases subside in time without treatment. In very mild cases, for example, affected skin stops itching and becomes crusted and dry in a few days; moderate cases usually run their course within 14 to 20 days. In dermatitis of routine severity, then, the effective treatment is one that assists the natural healing of the skin by keeping it clean, drying up broken blisters and relieving itching. Relatively simple medications such as "shake" lotions of calamine, which dries and soothes the skin, may be helpful. Some authorities recommend tepid baths in water containing cornstarch or oatmeal to relieve itching when the dermatitis is widely spread over the body. *The Medical Letter* reports that very hot water — at 120° or 130°F — has successfully relieved itching when dabbed on with a sponge or washcloth; some dermatologists, however, question the value of that treatment, since it tends to irritate the skin.

There is no conclusive evidence at this time that over-the-counter products are more effective, as a class, than those relatively simple — and inexpensive — treatments. Moreover, some persons are highly allergic to ingredients found in some over-the-counter creams and ointments; zirconia, tannic acid and antihistamines. As a result, many dermatologists feel that the danger of an allergic reaction to over-the-counter products far outweighs their theoretical virtues in soothing the itch of dermatitis.

Among prescription drugs, only the corticosteroid hormones, such as prednisone, are effective in treating the dermatitis. Most severely affected patients respond favorably, sometimes within a day or so. But corticosteroids must be administered under strict medical supervision. Oral dosage is effective, according to *The Medical Letter*. (But corticosteroids in cream or ointment forms for application to the skin have generally proved ineffective.)

Watch for the Leaf

Plants belonging to the poison-ivy family can be found in every state but Alaska and Hawaii. And poison ivy, as distinguished from poison oak and poison sumac, may appear under different guises in different localities or even within a single locality: sometimes as an upright shrub, bush or small tree, sometimes as a trailing plant that runs along the ground, sometimes as a climbing vine on fence, wall or tree. In whatever guise, the ivy is recognizable by its characteristic leaf, composed of three leaflets radiating from a single point of attachment. So the cautionary rhyme "Leaflets three, let it be" is worth heeding. Backyard poison ivy should be destroyed. If the growth is small, uprooting or grubbing out the plants may do the job. Protective clothing – trousers, long sleeves and gloves – should be worn, and suitable precautions taken in disposing of the plants. For large or for recurrent growths of the hardy weed, a treatment or series of treatments with a chemical herbicide may be needed. The chemicals are usually applied to best effect when the ivy's leaves are at their most luxuriant – June or July in most states. But herbicides must be handled with care, since some are harmful to humans and animals, to the soil and to harmless vegetation. . . .

Section V

First Aid for Problems of Heat and Cold

Three Heat Syndromes:
Exhaustion, Stroke and Cramps

How many people, accustomed to cool, air-conditioned homes and offices, will spend sweltering summer vacations and weekends on golf courses, beaches and tennis courts? How many will devote a hot humid Saturday to running the bases at a church picnic, or stand on a curb to watch a long Labor Day parade?

How many of these will collapse, victims of unaccustomed heat and humidity?

The three heat syndromes — exhaustion, stroke and cramps — are more prevalent today than ever, primarily because air conditioning has become a fact of life for so many people. While air conditioning brings relief, it also lessens the opportunity for the body to become naturally acclimated to heat — especially in short, concentrated exposures such as those described above. (The winter vacationer who leaves a cold climate for the tropics is equally susceptible.) This lessened resistance is compounded by the public's lack of knowledge about self-protection from environmental heat.

When a person is exposed to excessive heat, the result is peripheral vasodilatation, increased cardiac output and sweating. The heart rate increases, the blood pressure may drop slightly and, if physical exertion is undertaken, the heart may be unable to maintain proper blood pressure. If so, *heat exhaustion* — the commonest of the heat disorders — may follow.

Heat Stroke — the gravest of all heat disorders — may occur before heat exhaustion takes place, thereby blocking what is essentially a protective mechanism of the body. Heat stroke represents a failure of the heat-regulating mechanism of the body to adapt itself. Step-by-step, heat stroke results from exposure to excessive heat, and a high core temperature associated with a decrease and eventual halt in production of sweat. The body, deprived of its major defense against heat, stores more and more heat until cells in the vasomotor centers of the brain stem are damaged.

Heat Cramps are caused by an excessive loss of salt following strenuous exercise and profuse sweating. High external temperature is not a requisite; even in a cold environment, a heavily clothed person may suffer heat cramps if he is "out of shape" but is exercising violently (shoveling snow or climbing a steep hill, for example).

Fortunately, you can help people avoid these three heat disorders rather

By the editors of *Patient Care* in consultation with James R. Cade, M.D., H. Kay Dooley, M.D., and Kenneth Saer, M.D.

Adapted with permission from Miller and Fink Publishing Company, Darien, Conn.

easily. Simply remind them to properly acclimate themselves and to maintain a proper balance of salt and fluids during periods of heat stress. On the following pages, you will find some specific tips on prevention of heat problems, together with clues to the differential diagnoses and suggestions for treatment when a heat emergency does arise.

In preventing environmental heat disorders, acclimation and replacement of fluids and salts are vital steps.

To acclimate a person — whether to help him endure a heat wave at home or to adjust to an anticipated vacation in a hot climate — make sure that he understands the importance of promoting evaporation by exposing as much of his skin as possible to the air. Recommend loose-fitting clothes and brief him on protecting himself from the sun. One football team physician advises acclimatizing players each summer by having them work out for the first two weeks in tee shirts and shorts, before practicing in their loose-fitting cotton scrub suits.

If you know that an individual is going to a hot humid climate where he will be indulging in strenuous physical activity, or that he is an "air conditioned" individual who packs his weekends with golf or tennis, tell him to acclimate himself. He should get out in the heat for mild exercise as often as possible for short periods of time in advance. Start with 15-minute periods and gradually extend the period of exposure by 15-minute increments. Acclimation can usually be achieved within two weeks. The businessman who walks a few blocks every day to lunch, in preference to eating a sandwich at his desk, is better able to cope with a hot, active weekend. So is the housewife who walks to the store, in preference to telephoning for a delivery.

Caution both athletes and non-athletes to interrupt any physical activity periodically even if they are well acclimated. Anyone engaged in active exercise in the sun should pause for 5-10 minutes every half hour. This rule applies whether he is mowing his lawn or playing professional football.

The second step in preventing heat disorders is adequate replacement of fluids and salt.

Unfortunately, there have been two widespread misconceptions among the laity concerning both salt and fluids. Consequently, persons may, through ignorance, be misusing both.

Many men are in the habit of taking salt tablets during hot weather or strenous activity. Also, some individuals, whether or not they take salt tablets — firmly believe that they must never take *any* liquids while exercising; they fear that water will either make them nauseated or give them stomach cramps

Both of these practices — too much salt and too little fluid replacement — are dangerous. Many physicians believe that salt tablets should be taken only when prescribed, or under controlled conditions where the patient can be weighed before and after exercise.

How much salt and water is needed must be individually determined. If you feel that an individual's salt intake during meals is inadequate, three tablets daily (one half gram each, accompanied by a full glass of water) should suffice for most people — the 45-year-old executive weeding his garden, the farmer driving his combine, or the elderly patient who "feels the heat."

One program for young athletes calls for two one-half gram salt tablets with water 3-4 times a day; another stipulates 2-4 tablets before and after a game or practice. These athletes are weighed before and after exercise to determine fluid loss.

Some people become nauseated if they take salt tablets during physical activity; for such persons, try the flavored saline solutions which are available commercially and used by athletic directors and team physicians. The saline may be obtained through athletic suppliers and pharmacies, or direct from the manufacturers. Among them are: Gatorade (Stokley Van Camp Co., Indianapolis, Ind.); Take Five (Cramer Chemical, Gardner, Kansas); Sportade (Truett Labs., Dallas, Texas); and Trainade Salt Solution (School Health Supply, Addison, Ill.).

As a general rule, during physical activity, 6 ounces of saline solution (.1 percent salt, the body salt solution usually being .9 percent) is recommended. This will help compensate for any sudden loss of fluids and salt through exercise. A physically active person may need five quarts of fluid daily to replace that loss; the inactive, two quarts.

When the call comes — "Someone has collapsed from the heat" and is "writhing in agony" — is the caller trying to describe heat cramps, heat exhaustion, or a life-threatening heat stroke? Differentiating the disorders promptly is important since it will help determine your therapy — and in heat stroke, any delay may be fatal.

If the stricken "writhing" victim is a normally healthy individual who has been sweating profusely as a result of strenuous exercise, he may simply be having painful paroxysms from muscle cramps — not convulsions from heat stroke.

The attack may have occurred without warning, or the victim may have had premonitory symptoms of headache, vertigo, faintness and abdominal distress. He will be in excruciating pain, particularly in his leg and arm muscles and, perhaps, in his abdominal muscles as well. His skin will be gray, and cold and clammy to your touch. His pulse will be rapid, his blood pressure low and his temperature subnormal. He has been replacing fluids but not salt, so blood chemistries would show a low serum sodium and chloride.

In less severe cases of heat cramps, the victim will simply complain of tingling in his extremities and perhaps belly pain.

If you find the victim unconscious, rule out cramps. He may have collapsed from heat exhaustion or he may be exhibiting a sign of central nervous system disturbance due to heat stroke. Convulsions, often followed by unconsciousness and coma, are usually present in heat stroke. Your best clues in distinguishing between exhaustion and stroke are the feel of the person's skin and his temperature.

In heat exhaustion, the person's skin feels cold and clammy, his blood pressure is low and his temperature is subnormal or normal, since prostration develops prior to prolonged exposure. In heat stroke, sweating has stopped, the skin is fiery hot and dry, and the ... temperature is extremely high — temperatures as high as 112° have been recorded. A rectal temperature above 106° augurs for a grave prognosis. His blood pressure may be slightly elevated, and his repiration is weak and rapid.

In both types of heat syndrome the pulse will be rapid and evidence of circulatory collapse can be noted. The victim may appear to have had a myocardial infarction.

Some individuals with heat stroke may have had no apparent premonitory symptoms. However, close questioning of the family may reveal that the person complained of a diminution of sweating for a day or two preceding the attack. He also may have been irritable and unusually fatigued. For the few minutes immediately preceding their collapse, some heat stroke victims experience a sudden euphoria or exhibit confused, irrational behavior.

For heat cramps, generous quantities of oral saline solution usually result in cessation of paroxysms promptly. Some ... find salted lemonade (one teaspoonful of salt per quart) palatable. Also, insist on bed rest. Massage of the affected muscles is not helpful and may, in fact, aggravate the pain. It is rarely necessary to resort to hospitalization. ...

For heat exhaustion, move the patient into the shade, or preferably, a cool room. Remove his clothes and sponge him with wet, cool cloths and alcohol. Fanning will speed the cooling process. He may be uncomfortable if lying flat; support his head and shoulders. Since he has probably lost much salt and water, replace both with oral saline. He is apt to be nauseated from the attack and will not tolerate salt tablets. Heavy salting of food for the next few days and increased intake of fluids are adequate substitutes.

Victims of heat exhaustion do not usually require hospitalization. ... However, if there are signs of shock or impending heat stroke, immediate medical attention is indicated.

Heat stroke calls for immediate and heroic measures, including hospitalization as rapidly as possible. (Many physicians, in anticipation of the development of coagulative disorders, issue a blood donor alert at the same time they summon the ambulance.) While waiting for the ambulance, *the victim's temperature must be reduced without delay.* The length of exposure and the duration of high fever determine the outcome in most cases.

Move the victim to the coolest spot available, take off heavy outer clothing, apply cold wet towels and ice packs and start fanning him. Some authorities suggest wrapping the victim in a cold, wet sheet. The objective is to promote evaporation of moisture on the skin to help lower his temperature. If alcohol in any form is available, pour it on the victim.

In the ambulance, continue to cool the victim as best you can. Once in the emergency room of the hospital, the physician will probably give him an ice bath and cold water enema. Rectal temperatures should be taken often to ensure that his body temperature does not drop too fast, nor below 102°. If the temperature drops too rapidly, the resulting vasoconstriction will prevent diffusion of body heat and may cause convulsions. . . .

If a heat stroke victim survives beyond 24 hours, the prognosis is good. If he received prompt treatment and his temperature lowered quickly — within an hour — he will probably recover without neurological damage. However, any person who has had a heat stroke is permanently susceptible to the heat and should take every possible precaution when exposed to hot or humid weather.

HOT WEATHER HINTS FOR PATIENTS

If you become exposed to excessive heat this summer — or if you leave a cold climate next winter for a vacation in the tropics — your body may be unable to meet the demands of unaccustomed heat. If so, you may develop one of the following:

Heat cramps in your legs, arms and perhaps abdomen. These usually follow profuse sweating as a result of strenuous exercise and may be excruciatingly painful. If mild, you may only feel a tingling sensation in your extremities and perhaps a stomach ache.

Heat exhaustion. This may develop after just a short exposure to intense heat. You will feel exhausted and may collapse and lose consciousness.

Heat stroke. This may come on suddenly without warning or, a day or two preceding the attack, you may notice that you are perspiring less than usual, feel irritable and tired. When heat stroke occurs, sweating stops and your temperature soars. Convulsions, followed by unconsciousness and coma, are often present.

To condition yourself to the heat, follow these rules:

1. Expose as much of your skin to the air as possible. Wear loose fitting clothing.

2. Try to do the heaviest outdoor work in the cooler daytime hours — early morning or evening.

3. Don't avoid the heat entirely. Give yourself a chance to become acclimated by degrees. Spend 15 minutes in mild exertion the first day and gradually increase the time spent in daily exposure.

4. Always interrupt your physical exertion with a 5-10 minute rest period every half hour.

5. Drink water or salted lemonade (one teaspoonful of salt to a quart of lemonade) during your break.

6. Don't take salt tablets unless your physician prescribes them. Instead, salt your food heavily at mealtime.

7. Consult your physician at the first sign of trouble (excess or diminished sweating, fatigue, nausea, faintness, diarrhea, headache).

To avoid problems of sun exposure, follow these rules:

1. Take advantage of the moving sun. The time for burning is usually between 10 a.m. and 2 p.m. standard time. Avoid exposure during these hours and limit your exposure to 15-30 minutes.

2. Wear protective clothing and a broad-brimmed hat when in the midday sun. A tightly woven robe offers good protection at the beach.

3. Count swimming time and time under a beach umbrella as sunning time. About 85 percent of the burning rays of the sun go at least three feet below water surface. An umbrella will not prevent reflection of ultraviolet rays from sand and sky.

4. Use a good sunscreen. Several suntan lotions giving good protection are Solbar, Uval, Pabafilm, RVP, A-Fil and zinc oxide and titanium dioxide (many brands). If you use a cosmetic suntan lotion or pancake makeup, remember to keep a thick layer on. Don't be misled by "tanning" preparations containing dihydroxyacetone or iodine in baby oil. Your skin gets dyed — not tanned.

Use of Ice Water in the Treatment of Burns

E. B. Cunningham, M.D. and Jack L. Harris, M.D.

Relieving pain and minimizing the extent of tissue damage are two primary objectives of the emergency treatment of burns. Many methods have been employed, perhaps the most popular having been the old household remedy of applying butter or lard or a paste of sodium bicarbonate to the burned area. In industry, and where first aid kits are available, tannic acid and other forms of ointments have been used. None has been very effective in relieving the pain of an acute burn and the damage to tissues in the burned area has seemed to be unimpeded.

Recently, immersion in or application of ice water has been suggested as an emergency treatment for burns. In his recent review, Brown stated: "The application of cold to acute burns and scalds seems to be a very obvious procedure, but it is surprising how infrequently this method is used in practice. The use of cold decreases the edema and blistering, and the relief of pain and tenderness is quite remarkable in every case." (1)

Our experience tends to corroborate these statements. In fact, the results have been so good, particularly in limited burns of the face, neck and hands, that we routinely employ this technique.

All persons sustaining thermal or electric burns are brought to the medical department as promptly as possible. With chemical burns, sufficient delay is allowed for copious flushing under the emergency shower or any other convenient water source.

On his arrival at the medical department, the patient's clothing is removed and, whenever necessary, the burned area is gently cleansed with liquid soap and cold water. Then the burned area is immersed in water cooled with ice. When total immersion of the part is not possible, as with burns of the face, continuous cold compresses are applied.

As a rule, pain is relieved so promptly and completely that analgesic drugs are not required. If pain recurs when the part is removed from the ice water, immersion is repeated. The duration of immersion required ranges from 30 min. to 4 or 5 hr., depending upon the extent and the depth of the burn.

The cases described on the following page typify the results that have been obtained with this regimen.

Reprinted with permission from *Journal of Occupational Medicine*, May 1966, pp. 271-272.

Case Reports

Case 1 On Feb. 8, 1965, G.D., a 56-year-old white male, was inspecting a burner box at a coke plant. A leaking burner valve caused an explosion as a result of which the employee received what appeared to be first- and second-degree burns of the entire face and neck. He was seen at the medical department within 10 min. after the accident. The burn areas were cleansed with soap and cold water, and ice water compresses were applied to the burned areas. As the compresses warmed, they were changed. Relief of pain was almost instantaneous. The treatment was continued for approximately 3 hr., after which neomycin sulfate (0.5%) ointment was applied to the burned areas.

When seen again on the next day, there was no edema, erythema, or tenderness in the area of the burns. The patient continued to work and was discharged from treatment 10 days after the incident. The usual bleb formation and crusting that would ordinarily have been expected with this type of burn was not seen.

Case 2 On June 25, 1965, R.E., a 29-year-old white male was assisting in the repair of an acid line containing 50% sulfuric acid. As his assistant was breaking a union, acid sprayed out causing burns at the outer canthus of the right eye and what appeared to be third-degree burns of the right side of face, neck, and ear. The areas were treated by copious flushing with water followed by the application of ice water compresses. The latter were continued for approximately 2 hr., following which the areas were dressed with fluocinolone acetonide (0.25%) and neomycin sulfate (0.5%) cream. When the patient was seen on the following day, there was no blistering, edema, or tenderness. The areas were left open and the patient instructed to apply 0.5% neomycin sulfate ointment daily. He continued to work, and healing was pronounced complete, without scarring, in 13 days.

Case 3 On July 2, 1965, W.H., a 42-year-old white male, was splicing cable when the wrench he was using shorted across a 250-v d.c. line. There was a flash, and he sustained what appeared to be second-degree burns of all of the fingers, the thumb, and the thenar eminence of the right hand. When seen about 10 min. after the accident, the hand was placed in cold water, with almost instantaneous relief of pain. The immersion was continued for over 1 hr., and then the usual dressing applied. A large blister formed on the thumb and thenar eminence of the right hand but this healed without complication.

Case 4 On Oct. 14, 1965, E.M., a 38-year-old white male, was working with oxygen-acetylene welding equipment that caught fire. In attempting to put out the fire with a gloved hand, he sustained burns over the index finger, the web space between the index finger, and the thumb and the thenar eminence. The hand was immersed in ice water, with immediate relief of pain. This was continued for 2 hr., following which the hand was dressed with aureomycin gauze. Soon thereafter, the patient returned complaining of the pain. On reimmersion of the hand in ice water, the pain was immediately relieved. After 2 more hours (total immersion time, 4 hr.) he was able to remove his hand without pain. When seen the following day, there was only slight blistering of the web area between index finger and thumb.

Summary and Conclusions

The use of immersion in ice water or, when not practicable, the application of ice water compresses, has been most successful as an emergency treatment for burns of thermal, chemical, or electrical origin. In virtually every instance, it has provided instant and complete relief of pain and we have been uniformly delighted by the absence of edema, tenderness, and blistering that we had come to expect from such burns. We recommend, therefore, that it be adopted as first-aid treatment for burns involving limited portions of the body's surface.

Armco Steel Corp.
Middletown, Ohio

REFERENCES

1. Brown, C.R. "The Treatment of Burns by Cooling." *J. Abdom. Surg.* 2 (1960): 117.

Prevention and Treatment of Burns and Scalds

Richard Hurley, Ph.D.

Every year thousands of persons in the United States and throughout the world suffer painful injuries from various types of burns and scalds which all too often result in death or serious disfigurement to the victims. Many of these are children who must carry the burden of serious scarring for the rest of their lives. Many of the serious effects of burns and scalds could be prevented or their severity lessened through practicing a few simple preventive procedures. Also, through the practice of some rather basic first aid procedures the seriousness of burn injuries could be lessened when they do occur. It is to these purposes that this article is directed.

Degrees of Burns

Burn injuries are classified into three groups according to the depth of skin injury incurred. First degree burns are the most common and cause a reddening of the surface layer of the skin. Although first degree burns are extremely painful, they are usually not fatal unless large areas of the body are affected. Second degree burns are the next in frequency. With second degree burns the deeper layers of the skin are affected resulting in blistering due to the layers of the skin separating and pockets of body fluids accumulating. Burns of this degree can be considered quite dangerous if as little as ten percent of the total body surface is affected. A third degree burn results from total destruction of all the skin layers and can involve bones, muscles, and other body tissues. Any third degree burn must be considered extremely serious and will usually require long range hospitalization and reconstruction therapy.

Types of Burns

There are three general types of burns — thermal burns, chemical burns, and electric burns. Each type of burn imposes a different type of problem for the first-aider and will therefore be discussed separately.

It must be remembered that the purpose of first aid is to provide temporary emergency care to a burn victim until the services of a medical doctor can be obtained. This care should involve relieving pain, treating for shock, and preventing infection. As in all injuries, the first-aider must be extremely careful that what he does as first aid does not make the injury worse or interfere with the professional medical treatment the doctor will be giving later. A careful description of some acceptable first aid procedures will now be given.

The treatment for pain and shock is both relatively simple and in many ways related. The greatest concern in all treatment should be to prevent contamination. It is ironic that burn victims, whose injuries are relatively free from contamination, frequently die from septicemia or other forms of infection introduced through careless handling. Because the skin is partially or totally destroyed in second and third degree burns, much of the body's defense against infection is lost.

First Aid for First and Second Degree Burns

The first step in treating a victim of thermal burns of the first and second degree is immediate cooling of the injured area. Cool tap water will do very well for this. If the force of the water causes discomfort to the patient, a sterile pan or bowl can be used. If these are not available, a clean cloth or dressing can be immersed in cold water and used as a compress. Several new types of chemical cold packs are now available and should be included in a first aid kit. These will do an adequate job of temporarily cooling an area of the body if ice or cool water is not readily available. Ice packs can also be utilized if ice is available. A simple but effective ice pack can be prepared by dumping a tray of ice cubes in a towel or clean cloth and then, while holding the edges, striking the ice against a cupboard or wall several times. This does a good job of crushing the ice. Then place a clean cloth or small layer of plastic or Handi-wrap over the area and apply the ice pack. Then cover the complete area with a towel or similar covering. The method used is not really as important as the timing. Much of the trauma of a burn is due to increased capillary permeability and increased enzymatic action in the damaged tissues following a thermal injury. If the damaged tissue is not cooled, the tissue damage may continue for a prolonged period of time resulting in a much more serious injury. The immediate use of cold, by whatever method used, not only produces a rapid cessation of pain but can thus reduce the seriousness of the injury.

Treatment of injuries involving a large area of the body may require the use of a bathtub or other large container of water. All of the burned area should be placed in the cold water until the pain subsides. This may take several hours. A physician should be contacted and his instructions followed. After the burn has been properly cooled, sterile dressings or burn pads should be used to protect the injury while transporting to a hospital. If these are not available, a freshly laundered sheet will suffice.

Since swelling of fingers and hands may occur quite rapidly following a burn, it may be necessary to remove rings, bracelets, etc. Some situations may warrant the cutting away of clothing fragments from around an injured area. If this is attempted, one must be extremely careful to not touch or to allow the clothing to come in contact with the damaged tissue. Generally, this could better be done under the more sterile conditions of a physician's office since some tissue debridement may be necessary also.

Salves, ointments, and other "home grown," topical applications are of questionable value in treating burns and should be avoided unless a physician recommends their use.

First Aid for Third Degree Burns

Problems encountered from victims of third degree burns are much more serious. There is very little the first-aider can do except keep the wound as clean as possible, treat the victim for shock, and get medical treatment for the injured as soon as possible. Cooling with water, as previously discussed for first and second degree burns, should not be attempted. In many cases the pain may not be as great since many of the pain receptor cells and sensory neurons are destroyed by the injury. Clothing which is still smoldering should be cut away and then the complete burned area should be covered with a sterile burn dressing if available. If sterile dressings are not available, then freshly laundered sheets, tightly woven towels, or similar materials can be used. The wound may be left exposed while dressings are sterilized by ironing or passing over an open flame. It is essential that the materials used be as clean as possible. The dressing should then be bandaged snugly in place but not so tightly that it impairs circulation. Enough bandaging should be used to shut out the air as much as possible. This will help reduce the pain. Cotton or very loose nap materials should not be used as a dressing since the fibers tend to transfer to the wound and contaminate it.

In all burn injuries immediate treatment should begin as soon as possible to prevent the onset of shock. This should begin by keeping the injured person lying down. This may not be possible while administering the water-cooling procedures previously discussed. However, the victim should be kept as calm and quiet as possible. They should be given constant reassurance that their needs are being met. Body heat should be maintained by keeping the injured person covered. The amount of covering should be regulated to maintain body heat but not elevate it. The victim's comfort is the primary concern.

First Aid for Chemical Burns

Chemical burns may result from contact with strong acids, alkalies, or other chemicals. The burning will continue as long as the offending material is in contact with the skin. Therefore, this should be our immediate concern. Clothing should be removed as rapidly as possible and showering or washing with a hose or other source of water should begin immediately. If the chemical has entered the eye, it must be flushed out completely. Speed is essential since many chemicals can do very serious damage in a short period of time. The eye can be placed directly under a faucet allowing a small stream of water to irrigate and wash out the eye thoroughly. All cases of eye burns from chemicals should be seen by a medical specialist as soon as possible to avoid permanent damage.

Most attempts to neutralize chemical burns are relatively unsuccessful and all too often are responsible for further injury. For this reason this practice is discouraged unless, as in the case of many work areas where chemicals are frequently used, the neutralizing agent is known and procedures for its usage have been previously discussed and outlined. After all traces of the chemical have been washed from the body, sterile dressings should be applied and then the injured person transported to a doctor or hospital.

First Aid for Electrical Burns

Causes of electric burns are many and varied and may be accompanied by associated problems such as cessation of breathing and heart stoppage. Any attempts at first aid must be preceded by the determination of the source of the electricity and its elimination if possible. If the power source cannot be shut off and the victim is still in contact with a wire or other source, extreme caution must be used. The first-aider must never use his hands or any other material capable of conducting electricity. A dry stick or similar object should be used to reduce contact with the source of electricity, then move the victim several feet away before treatment is begun. Be especially careful that onlookers or yourself do not accidentally contact the live wire or electrical source. Immediate treatment should then be started to restore breathing if stopped. After vital signs have been restored, the burns should be treated by the method previously discussed, followed by transporting the victim to a physician.

Prevention of Burn Injuries

All burn injuries are serious and in most cases could have been prevented. Although some serious burn accidents occur at work, in cars, and away from the home, most occur in the home and are usually the result of someone's carelessness. All persons would do well to re-evaluate their personal practices to see if they are inviting a burn injury to themselves, a loved one, or others who visit their homes.

Every homeowner should conduct periodic inspections of his home to see if fire hazards can be detected. Such things as a pile or container of soiled rags left over from the last paint job can spontaneously ignite and start a fire. Frayed wires and cords could cause a serious electric burn or start a fire. Many volatile substances such as kerosene, solvents, paints, etc., require special care in storing. Most fire departments will assist you in inspecting your home free of charge if requested. At the same time they could make recommendations concerning the location of fire extinguishers, hoses, etc.

Perhaps more important would be an examination of our own safety practices. Do we smoke in bed? Do we use appliances and equipment the way they were designed to be used? Do we always keep pot handles turned in away from the reaching hands of children? Do we keep matches and other sources of flame away from children? And, finally, do we give our children the training they need? For example, are regular fire drills held? Have we taught our children how to roll to put out a fire in their clothes? These questions may seem rather simple yet their answers could determine whether you or your child will be the victim of a serious burn accident.

REFERENCES

1.   Cole, Warren H. and Puestow, Charles B. *First Aid – Diagnosis and Manage-ment*. New York: Appleton-Century-Crofts, 1965.
2.   Henderson, John. *Emergency Medical Care*. New York: McGraw-Hill Book Company, 1969.
3.   Monafo, William W. *The Treatment of Burns*. St. Louis: Warren H. Green Inc., 1971.
4.   "First Aid Therapy for Burns – Cool It!" *Clinical Pediatrics,* December 1970.
5.   Potthoff, Carl J. "First Aid – Clinical Injuries." *Today's Health,* December 1970.
6.   Shaw, Bernice L. "Current Therapy for Burns." *RN*, March 1971.

First Aid for Cold Injuries

Brent Q. Hafen, Ph.D.

Every year hundreds of Americans sustain permanent cold injuries from frostbite. The results range from hypersensitivity to cold to that of amputation because of tissue death. It has been suggested by numerous medical personnel that most of these instances of frostbite, excluding those situations in which accident and injury complicate the problem, could be prevented. However, prevention can only be accomplished by educating the public in early care first aid. Recent work concerning the pathogenesis of cold injury suggests that the most important advance in first aid measures for the general public is the technique of rapid rewarming. Rapid rewarming, however, is not recommended when body tissues have been thawed and then refrozen. Even though frostbite is more of a problem in the northern sections of the United States, persons in the southern United States are often more prone to frostbite than those in the North. This is probably due to the fact that those individuals raised in the southern states often do not have the knowledge nor the opportunity to adjust to the cold. It is interesting to note that blacks usually require a longer period of time to adjust to the cold than do whites.

The great variety of first aid measures that have existed throughout the years for the problem of frostbite is probably the result of the lack of information of the pathophysiology of this particular form of cold injury.

What Is Frostbite?

"True frostbite means frozen tissues. Crystals of ice form between the cells. As the crystals grow in size they draw water from the cells damaging them. Nerves, muscles, and blood vessel tissues are most susceptible to frostbite." (1) Depending on various circumstances, anyone who is exposed to temperatures below 32°F is a candidate for frostbite, which may result in a partial or total freezing of certain body tissues. Figure 1 depicts some of the circumstances and conditions of exposure in the pathophysiology of frostbite (2). We find that frostbite more commonly occurs in the peripheral areas of the body: feet, hands, ears, and nose in that order. This freezing may extend up the arms and legs as exposure is prolonged. When the body is chilled, the principal effect is a constriction of the blood vessels, particularly in the extremities. This, of course, reduces the skin temperature, which results in a conservation of body heat. A combination of extreme cold and severe vessel constriction can make it so circulation may almost totally cease in localized areas. As the circulation becomes severely impaired, the sensation of cold or related pain is lost and, as the tissues

FIGURE 1
PATHOPHYSIOLOGY OF FROSTBITE

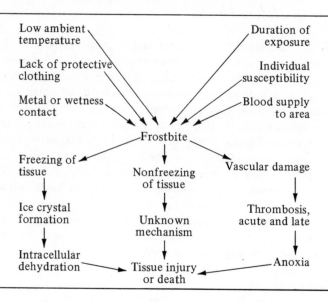

actually begin to freeze, the frozen area enlarges and becomes deeper; this is the point at which the ice crystals actually form between the cells and then grow by drawing water from within the cells. This may result in physical injury by the ice crystals as well as dehydration which, of course, would affect the biochemical balance inside the cell.

Cold injury is more likely to occur at temperatures of 32°F and lower when high wind is blowing because heat is more rapidly taken from the body. This can be seen from Figure 2, the wind-chill factor chart (3). It is evident that frostbite potential increases with the wind velocity.

Persons who have poor circulation, who are in a state of exhaustion, who are extremely nervous and excitable, and also those who sweat profusely have less resistance to cold; therefore the potential for frostbite is greater. It is also important to realize that altitude may have an effect on the frostbite potential. The higher the altitude the less available oxygen is for the body, which may result in hypoxia or a shortage of oxygen for the tissues, and this increases the susceptibility to frostbite. Moisture also increases the frostbite potential along with incidences of coming in contact with steel, gasoline, liquid oxygen, carbon dioxide, Freon, and other such liquids and industrial gases. Although injuries sustained by contact with these types of substances are often referred to as chemical burns, the body tissues are actually frozen.

FIGURE 2
WIND CHILL FACTOR CHART

Estimated wind speed (in mph)	Actual Thermometer Reading (°F.)											
	50	40	30	20	10	0	-10	-20	-30	-40	-50	-60
	EQUIVALENT TEMPERATURE (°F.)											
calm	50	40	30	20	10	0	-10	-20	-30	-40	-50	-60
5	48	37	27	16	6	-5	-15	-26	-36	-47	-57	-68
10	40	28	16	4	-9	-24	-33	-46	-58	-70	-83	-95
15	36	22	9	-5	-18	-32	-45	-58	-72	-85	-99	-112
20	32	18	4	-10	-25	-39	-53	-67	-82	-98	-110	-124
25	30	16	0	-15	-29	-44	-59	-74	-88	-104	-118	-133
30	28	13	-2	-18	-33	-48	-63	-79	-94	-109	-125	-140
35	27	11	-4	-20	-35	-51	-67	-82	-98	-113	-129	-145
40	26	10	-6	-21	-37	-53	-69	-85	-102	-116	-132	-148
(Wind speeds greater than 40 mph have little additional effect.)	LITTLE DANGER (for properly clothed person). Maximum danger of false sense of security.			INCREASING DANGER Danger from freezing of exposed flesh.			GREAT DANGER					

Signs and Symptoms of Frostbite

The most noticeable early warning symptoms of frostbite are whiteness of the frozen part, especially in ears and nose. The frozen part becomes hard with little or no feeling. This may be preceded by a tingling sensation and a numbness. The tingling sensation would be that characterized by the typical "pins and needles" feeling. This is then followed by numbness. The affected part may then become painful with a red flush to the skin. If freezing continues, the affected part becomes quite hard with the loss of all sensation, and the skin then becomes a dead white, gray, or gray-yellow color. Generally then, a frostbitten victim will usually complain that first the affected part was painful and then numb. The frozen part remains free of pain while frozen.

The severity of the cold injury is often classified according to the extent of tissue damage: first degree frostbite usually results in injury to surface skin somewhat like a sunburn. A redness with a feeling of warmth, swelling, burning, and tingling sensations without the formation of blisters may be present. However, there is usually no tissue loss. In second degree frostbite, blisters are usually produced. However, the appearance is similar to that of first degree. The blisters may appear anywhere from minutes to hours after the cold injury. This may be accompanied by an undue redness of the skin on rewarming. Edema or swelling may also be present. In third degree frostbite injury there is usually damage to the deep tissues and much of the frozen part may be lost. The full thickness of skin injury is usually present with swelling in the early stages — blisters are usually absent. This may result in early necrosis and possibly gangrene but not necessarily with the loss of the affected part. In fourth degree injury there is usually complete necrosis with loss of the part, which may affect not only the skin but muscle and possibly bone. There is usually no blister and no swelling. It is important to realize that unless proper prevention and first aid measures are taken, severe frostbite may result in amputation in very severe cases and in less severe may leave the victim hypersensitive to cold for the rest of his life. It should further be realized that during and following the thawing of a frostbitten part of the body the area is often painful and swollen. The tenderness and swelling usually reduce over a period of several days. As thawing occurs in minor cases the affected part may appear to be red with the possibility of blistering and skin peeling. In more severe cases or in situations where proper first aid has not been rendered, the affected part may still have a dull or ashen color which may later turn black. Even in mild cases of frostbite the appearance during the stage of blistering is often frightening. It is important to remember that this appearance may be disturbing even in mild cases; therefore the victim should be encouraged and should not be allowed to become alarmed.

The Prevention of Frostbite

It is obvious that prevention is the best protection against frostbite. It would then follow that everything should be done to conserve the body's heat and nothing should be done that would diminish the body's heat production. Knowing what type of clothing to wear on days when the temperature is low is extremely important. On cold days several layers of loose fitting, lightweight clothing should be worn. In that way if a person becomes engaged in some type of strenuous activity or exercise, he can remove the layers of clothing as needed to prevent perspiring and subsequent chill.

The clothing that is worn on days of this type should be tightly woven and water repellent. However, it is suggested that waterproof clothing not be used since it tends to hold moisture in, and in cases of perspiration this would increase the body heat loss. Rather the clothing should be of a nature that the outer garments are windproof and the inner garments are the "waffle" or knit underclothing that tends to trap air and hold the warm air close to the body. The hands should be protected by mittens instead of gloves. That way the fingers keep each other warm. If possible the coat or parka that is worn should have a hood that is large enough to cover the face and mouth if necessary. The shoes or boots should be worn with a lightweight cotton sock next to the skin and a heavy woolen or synthetic sock covering the lighter stocking. The shoes or boots should be well broken in, should be large enough to fit comfortably, and should not be so tight as to constrict circulation and add to frostbite danger. In fact, all type of tight clothing or garters that may restrict circulation should be avoided.

As previously mentioned, moisture is a factor in frostbite because moisture tends to conduct heat and, if you are out in the cold and wet, the heat tends to be conducted away from the body. Therefore, it is important to avoid any unnecessary overexertion and excessive perspiration. If you find yourself with increased perspiration, your activity should be reduced and/or one of the outer lighter garments should be removed. It is important to keep clothing dry from outside moisture as well as from inside perspiration. It is also important to avoid contact of the bare skin with cold metal or gasoline. Gasoline tends to take on the temperature of the surrounding area and cools the skin by evaporation.

Another factor to remember is that inadequate calorie intake or physical exhaustion may reduce the body's energy reserves to such a level that the body temperature can no longer be maintained. Therefore, if a person realizes that he is going to be working out in the cold weather for any period of time, it is important that he have an adequate intake of food so enough calories are made available to the body that the body temperature can be maintained.

One never knows when there is going to be an emergency situation such as a stalled car or an auto accident. For this reason it is suggested that you carry heavy clothing and shoes in your car. And if your auto stalls in cold weather some distance from help, you'll be prepared to safely seek help. However, if adequate clothing is not available, it may be safer to stay at the scene of the accident or at the stalled car. Help is more likely to find an individual if he remains close to his vehicle. If there is no adequate shelter, even if you are properly dressed you should keep moving by walking and moving the arms and legs to help keep the circulation up and reduce the potential chance of frostbite. Don't forget, the wind has a marked effect on how rapidly the body loses heat. Accordingly it may be necessary to dress comparatively well on a warm winter day because of the rapid rate at which the heavy wind is blowing your body heat away. Conversely, lighter outer clothing only may be needed on a colder day when the wind and air is still and allows the body to conserve heat longer. It seems then the best way to prevent frostbite is to be prepared for the cold, to dress for the cold, and to use common sense when working or playing in the cold. Not just the cold by the thermometer but also the conditions that relate to frostbite such as the windchill factor and moisture.

Should First Aid Be Rendered?

Through the years a variety of first aid treatments for frostbite have been used, and many have been known to be ineffective and even harmful. For example, rubbing the frozen part with snow or ice for the purpose of restoring circulation is particularly bad. The frozen tissue may be bruised and gangrene may even result. In past years slow rewarming of the affected part has also been recommended, but this is no longer advocated. The frozen part should be treated with gentleness and should not be rubbed or massaged. It is also important to remember that a frostbite victim should not be given tobacco or alcoholic beverages. Alcohol dilates the blood vessels, bringing them closer to the surface of the skin with increased blood flow, which temporarily produces a feeling of warmth but eventually results in an increased loss of heat. Tobacco use should also be avoided because it constricts the blood vessels, thereby reducing needed blood circulation to the tissue area that is being threatened by frostbite. It seems then that the biggest problems in past first aid treatment have been that of slow rewarming, unnecessary rough treatment by massage, and exercise with the idea of restoring circulation.

All frostbite regardless of how mild or severe should be seen by a physician. Help should be sought immediately. In some circumstances, if there is a possibility that the victim can reach a doctor or a hospital within a short period of time, even up to several hours, perhaps the best first aid treatment would be gentle handling and protection of the frozen part. If the affected part thaws and then becomes refrozen there is a possibility that the injury may become more severe than if it was not thawed at all. Medical treatment is not only needed but important because in many cases control of severe pain is required. Antibiotics and/or antitetanus injections may be needed if the skin is broken.

What To Do If First Aid Treatment Is Necessary

The thawing of the affected body tissue as soon as possible is of major importance in first aid for frostbite. However, rapid rewarming should not be attempted until there can be no further chilling or until the victim has reached a shelter or place where his entire body can be kept warm during and after the rendering of first aid and from which he can be removed for medical treatment without the possibility of refreezing the affected part. Rapid rewarming is a preferred first aid treatment with the exception, however, of when the part has been frozen, thawed, and then refrozen. As previously suggested this problem can be avoided by not thawing the part until the person either reaches a hospital, physician, or shelter in which proper rewarming can take place. If necessary, initiate treatment for shock.

Rapid rewarming can be accomplished by immersion in a large container, preferably a bathtub or a whirlpool if available. Use water between body temperature (98.6°F) and 105°F. Water any hotter than 105°F should be avoided. A thermometer should be used to continually monitor the temperature of the water, and as it cools additional hot water should be added.

In addition to rewarming, the affected part should be protected from further injury; therefore, do not allow it to touch a hot container or do not attempt rapid rewarming by placing frozen parts in a warm oven or close to an open fire. Hot, moist treatment is the best within the aforementioned temperature zone and, if a whirlpool or a large container or bathtub is not available, second best would be a wet towel. The towel should be constantly changed to maintain the recommended temperature level and should be placed on the frozen part gently with no rubbing. If a thermometer is not available to continually gage the water temperature, the first-aider should check to see that the water feels mild and comfortably warm to his touch. For the purposes of rewarming, the affected extremity should be stripped of all clothing and any types of constricting bands or objects. It will take approximately 20-45 minutes to thaw out a frozen part in water that is about body temperature. Once the part is warm, the victim should be encouraged to gently move the affected part to aid in the restoration of circulation. However, if the affected parts are the feet or legs, the person should not be allowed to walk. Following rewarming the victim must be kept warm, he may be given warm liquids to drink, and if the affected part is painful, aspirin could be given. If blisters form, they should not be disturbed and bandages, ointments, and other such substances should not be put on the frostbitten part. The victim should be seen by a physician as soon as possible.

What If a Physician Is Not Available?

Under some circumstances, it may be necessary to follow immediate first aid with treatment that may require several days or weeks due to the inaccessibility of a doctor or hospital. The victim needs bed rest and should remain in bed until all swelling subsides and sores are healed. The affected area should be cleansed with an antiseptic soap and warm water. Subsequent care should be treatment as a burn and should be directed toward preventing infection. Cleanliness of the frostbitten area is extremely important. Only soft sterile materials should be used to dress the frostbitten area. However, many physicians are now recommending that dressings not be applied. Sterile cotton may be put between the toes or fingers if necessary to prevent them from sticking together. It is extremely important that the victim be handled gently and protectively.

A first-aider should never attempt any further treatment of a frostbitten victim than the basic emergency steps unless absolutely necessary.

REFERENCES

1. Maxwell, Edward. "First Aid Treatment for Frostbite." *Today's Health*, Vol. 43, January 1965.
2. Knize, D.M.; Weatherly-White, R.C.; Paton, B.C.; Owens, J.C. "Prognostic Factors in the Management of Frostbite." *Journal of Trauma* 9(1969)749.
3. Boswick, John A. Jr.; Golding, Michael R.; Sumner, David S.; Weatherly-

White, R.C. "Frostbite: New Approaches Plus the Best of the Old." *Patient Care*, 15 November 1971.

4.   Owens, J. Cuthbert. "Treatment of Cold Injuries." *Postgraduate Medicine*, September 1970.

5.   Erven, Lawrence W. *First Aid and Emergency Rescue*. Glencoe Press, 1970.

6.   Wilkerson, James A., ed. *Medicine for Mountaineering*. Seattle, 1969.

First Aid for Common Medical Emergencies

Common Emergencies

Ray A. Petersen, M.H.Ed.

There are several conditions that suggest medical emergencies. Two key conditions are pain and unconsciousness. This chapter deals primarily with these two; however, fever, vomiting, and diarrhea are also involved. Sometimes they occur together and sometimes separately. Frequently they can be handled by home care, but at times they require emergency medical care. In the meantime the skill in administering the proper first aid may save lives and prevent permanent injury and unnecessary suffering. The following deals with a considerable number of illnesses or abnormalities in which one and usually more of these conditions are found. Some of these do not occur often enough to be truly called common; but when they do occur, they constitute an emergency. Others are fairly common but hardly constitute an emergency. Put together, they comprise a significant area of first aid.

The various cases of aches and pains will be considered first, starting with the head and working downward. Then those emergencies that may cause unconsciousness will be considered. Vomiting, diarrhea, and fever will be dealt with as they apply.

Pain

Pain is nature's warning that something is wrong. It may be a blessing because it gets the patient to the doctor for treatment. The source of pain in an accident may be obvious; the cause of pain in disease and illness may be more difficult to determine.

Pain is produced by irritation of the sensory nerve. Pain varies among different people, some are more sensitive than others. Pain varies with cause. Pain may be described as cutting, gnawing, boring, burning, throbbing, piercing, etc. A description of the type of pain and its point of origin may help determine its cause. The origin of the pain may be misleading because some conditions produce referred pain; the cause may be in one area while the pain is in another. The problem of referred pain emphasizes the danger of self-diagnosis and self-treatment, and the need for seeking medical attention. Some pain is also psychogenic or entirely mental.

The occasional mild pain may suggest simple home care, but when pain is severe or continues for more than two or three hours, or when it comes back again, it should be investigated by a physician. It may be an emergency requiring immediate medical or surgical attention, or it may be a chronic condition that can only be relieved by a physician. In the meantime, first aid measures can help relieve the pain and reduce the severity of the condition. A person's life or well-being may rest with the first-aider's ability to recognize the emergency and secure medical help.

Aches and Pain of the Head

Headaches

An aching head or a head pain is a symptom rather than a condition itself. It can suggest different underlying causes such as mental or emotional disturbances, eyestrain, hunger, constipation, indigestion, kidney disease, menstruation, onset of infectious disease, fever, fatigue, tension, allergy, sinusitis, high blood pressure, alcohol "hangover," or brain tumor.

Migraine is a severe type of headache. It may be accompanied by nausea, dizziness, chills, flushing, fluid retention, weakness, and signs of shock. Although its cause is not known it seems to be tied in with emotional problems. Good health practices — mental and physical — will help free the victim from suffering. Anyone prone to migraines should discuss the plan of treatment with his physician so that prescription remedies may be on hand in advance. Migraines can be stopped or lessened if medications are taken at the first appearance. The migraine sufferer should lie down in a quiet dark room with cold applications at the base of his skull and on his forehead. A doctor should be consulted.

The tension headache is less severe, but more common. Many forms of pain relievers and tranquilizers help relieve the symptoms of the tension; however, some may produce undesirable or dangerous effects, especially when one is driving a car. Aspirin is one of the safest to use and probably one of the most effective. One or two tablets are all that is required for the average person with the average headache. If this does not provide relief, a physician should be consulted.

If the headache comes on with sudden intensity, if it reoccurs with increasing intensity, if it is a different kind of headache than one has had before, or if it is not relieved by previously effective medications, you should consult your doctor to make sure that there is no serious underlying cause. Prolonged self-treatment is unwise.

Earache

There are many causes of earache. An earache resulting from a sudden change in altitude may be relieved by frequent yawning or chewing gum. Water in the ear may cause temporary discomfort. Pain most often results from infection in the ear. It is usually a secondary infection which has spread from the nose or throat through the eustachian tube. Forcefully blowing the nose during a cold may force infectious material into the ear. Forceful application of nasal sprays or douches may do the same. Infection in the ear can be very serious because of the possible loss of hearing and the proximity of the ear and the brain. An earache should always be suspected if a child is ill and has a fever. The child may pull his ear or turn his head frequently.

A sore throat is usually not an emergency but should be taken seriously and should be reported to your doctor. As mentioned, the infection can spread to the ears or cause some other secondary infection. A sore throat may lead to a serious disease such as rheumatic fever. Your doctor may advise the use of a commercial or a salt water gargle. For salt water, gargle for five minutes every hour with a solution of 1 teaspoon of table salt to one-half glass of hot water.

Eye Pain

Complaints that the eye itches should be taken seriously, and if it persists a physician should be contacted. Inflammation of the eye can be due to many causes. Pink eye is highly contagious and is prevalent during childhood; precautions should be taken to prevent its spread. The eye is inflamed and has a brilliant pink color. The eye may be swollen and a yellowish discharge tends to dry in crusts on the lids. One should be kept quiet and isolated. Cold compresses are helpful in relieving pain and inflammation.

Vernal catarrh is not infectious, but is an allergy due to sensitivity to pollens, dust, dyes, or animal dander. Symptoms consist of inflammation, bloodshot appearance, itching eyelids, and a watery discharge. The treatment consists of avoiding the offending agent and applying anti-allergy drugs.

A sty is an infection in a tiny gland or hair follicle along the margin of the eyelid. The center turns yellow and may discharge drops of pus. Wet compresses as warm as the victim can stand, applied for 20 minutes every three or four hours, give comfort and hasten recovery.

A small foreign body in the eye will cause inflammation. Do not rub the eye. Wash your hands before examining or touching the eye. Have the person assume a comfortable position with his head resting firmly against a wall, a bed, or other solid surface. Bring the upper eyelid down over the lower and hold it there for a few moments while the victim looks upwards. This will cause tears to flow, often washing out the foreign body. If this does not work, gently lift the eyelids back and try to see the object. First pull the lower lid down and have the victim look upward. If the foreign body is not revealed, invert the upper eyelid by holding the lashes and turning the lid inside out over the index finger of the opposite hand or over a cotton swab and have the victim look down. If you can see it, try to lift it by touching it lightly with a moistened sterilized cotton swab or the moistened corner of a handerchief. If this doesn't work it may be flushed out with a medicine dropper filled with water at body temperature. If this does not work either, take the person to a doctor. (Do not try to remove an object imbedded in the eye.) In the meantime, bandage both eyes shut to keep them from moving and causing further irritation.

Many chemicals can cause damage when they get into the eye if prompt and correct first aid action is not taken. Hold the head under a faucet or over a drinking fountain so that a stream of cold water flushes out the eye. The stream should not be forceful enough to damage the eye. Another approach is to have him lie down with his head tilted slightly upwards. Gently pour water from a glass or other container into the inner corner of the eye near the nose so that it flows across the eye and out at the outer edge of the eye. After the chemical has been thoroughly washed out of the eye, put several drops of clean olive oil, castor oil, or mineral oil into the eye. Then cover it with a sterile gauze compress and bandage it into place. Then call a doctor.

Toothache

Toothache is the reaction of irritated nerve endings within the tooth to decay or accident. It may hurt when a particle of food or hot or cold water enters the cavity, or the pain may be caused by inflammation at the root end of the tooth. Consult a dentist as soon as possible. In the meantime, some temporary relief may be obtained as follows: If there is a cavity in the aching tooth, clean it out by picking at it gently with a toothpick wrapped at the point with a whisp of sterile cotton, or rinse it vigorously with tepid water. Then saturate a tiny bit of sterile cotton with oil of cloves and pack it gently into the cavity or place it next to the cavity. Be careful not to spill the oil of cloves on the tongue or inside the mouth for it will burn.

A normal dose of aspirin may lessen the pain, but never place an aspirin tablet on the tooth or the gum tissue surrounding the tooth. Holding a mouthful of ice water in the mouth gives relief in some instances. Other times hot packs or heating pads applied to the cheek will give some slight relief. Lying down tends to increase pain, so sit up in a comfortable chair or prop yourself up in bed.

When a filling is lost or a tooth is broken off, chew some paraffin or candle wax with some strands of sterile cotton and use this to cover the jagged edges of the tooth until you can get to a dentist. If in an injury to the face a tooth is loosened or knocked out, apply ice packs to the injured side of the face and go to the dentist immediately. If a tooth is knocked out, keep it clean and *moist* — perhaps you could wrap it in a clean wet cloth or put it in a cup of water — and immediately take it with you to a dentist. Dentists have sometimes been successful in replanting teeth.

Skin Disorders

Boils and Pimples

Boils are a type of skin disorder that may be painful. The chief danger from boils and pimples occurs when they are located around the upper lip, nose, or eyes. The danger is that the infection may spread to the nervous system. Infection in this area requires medical attention. Do not squeeze any boil or pimple; to do so may cause the infection to spread. Hot moist packs will hasten the healing. A draining boil should be kept clean and covered with a dressing. A doctor can lance a boil and this aids the healing and reduces the pain. He can also give medications that will help. If a red or blue streak occurs along the arm or leg or if lumps or swelling occurs at the lymphatic nodes, contact your doctor.

Allergy

Allergies are usually not particularly painful, but they are very irritating. They can also be alarming when a person doesn't know what is causing it. Allergy of the membrane of the respiratory system can be very dangerous. An allergy is an abnormal tissue reaction to normally harmless substances. It can range from mild itching to hives, to hay fever, to asthma. The cause may range from food, medicine, and stings to emotional factors. With some people, death can result from a severe reaction to bee stings. If there is a tingling, itching, or swelling of the lips, tongue, or the inside of the mouth, call your doctor at once. Do not take any food, medicine, or drinks, (except water) until the doctor tells you to do so. Do not take a hot bath for it may aggravate it.

Hives

Hives are slightly elevated pinkish patches or welts that suddenly develop on the skin. Relief from hives can be obtained from cool applications of bicarbonate of soda or epsom salts. Calamine lotion will also help. A doctor can prescribe other medications and can help you find the cause of the allergy so that it can be prevented.

Breathing Difficulty

Croup

Croup in children and asthma in children and adults may cause difficulty in breathing. Sometimes emergency action is necessary to maintain breathing. Babies and children are sometimes affected by an infection causing spasms or swelling of the larnyx and trachea and bronchi. This hinders breathing. Difficulty in breathing often panics a child, for he feels that he is suffocating.

Call a physician and follow his directions. Reassure the child and keep him warm and in bed. Breathing may be easier in a sitting-up position. Give the child steam inhalation. If you have a commercial vaporizer, follow the manufacturer's instructions. Steam from boiling water in a tea kettle or pan may be funneled with a cone or folded paper so the child can breathe it while in bed. A tent-like canopy can be used to keep the steam in the area. The steam should not come in direct contact with the patient. Be careful not to spill the hot water. Steam can also be produced temporarily by running a large stream of hot water in the bathtub. The patient can lean over the tub and inhale the steam.

Asthma

An allergic reaction may be an asthmatic attack with difficulty in breathing. An allergic reaction may be to foreign substances such as dust, pollen, cosmetics, medicine, food, or insect stings, or to emotional factors or heart conditions. Swelling or edema at the base of the tongue or in the bronchial tubes makes breathing labored, wheezing, and accompanied by frequent coughing. The lips may be bluish.

Call a physician promptly. Be calm and try to reassure the victim. Fresh air or a sitting-up position will facilitate breathing. Steam inhalation may be helpful. The best procedure is prevention by avoiding the foreign substances one is sensitive to.

Choking

Suffocation is the most frequent cause of accidental death to children under one year of age and occasionally results in death of adults. A foreign body in the throat or windpipe may cause choking. Usually if the victim can remain calm and relax he can cough it up, but if this does not occur you must work fast. First, get the victim in position. If it is an infant, hold it by its ankles letting the head hang straight down. If it is a child, hold him face down across your lap with his head and shoulders hanging lower than your lap. If it is an adult, have the patient bend forward or lie across a chair, bed, or table with his head and shoulders hanging over the side. If you can't do this, roll him on one side on the floor, open his mouth, and pull the tongue forward. Then hit him hard with your hand between the shoulder blades to try to dislodge the object. If the object is removed but breathing is not spontaneous, start mouth-to-mouth artificial respiration. If you cannot remove the obstruction within one minute, start mouth-to-mouth artificial respiration to try to force air past the object.

Chest Pain

Pain in the chest should receive prompt medical attention. Such pain may come from so many causes — some serious and others not so serious — it is difficult even for a physician to determine the cause.

Pleurisy

Chest pains that come on gradually and that are accompanied by a cold or coughing or fever may be from pneumonia or pleurisy. These pains may be made worse by breathing. They make breathing "catch" or make the sufferer hold his breath. If these chest pains come on suddenly they are probably due to a strained chest or back muscle or from an injured rib. Call a doctor if the pains or breathing difficulty persists. Find a comfortable bed position and keep warm. This may be a sitting-up or a semi-reclining position. Take aspirin for pain.

Angina

Angina pectoris is an uncomfortable sensation of pressure, tightness, and pain usually in the front of the chest and may extend down the left arm. It is a sign that the heart muscle is not getting enough oxygen. It should be reported to your doctor for it may be a forerunner of a heart attack.

Heart Attacks

A pressure or squeezing pain in the chest, associated with pain in the shoulders and neck and radiating into the arms, may be a symptom of a heart attack. Nausea, vomiting, a cold sweat, and difficulty in breathing may be present. One's color may turn pale. This is not the heartburn-type pain.

If the pain is persistent or severe, a doctor should be called. Keep the patient warm and have good ventilation. It is best to lie down, but if there is a shortness of breath, a sitting position may be more comfortable. Protect the victim from exertion and emotional strain. Do not try to move him. If he has had heart attacks before he may have some medication. Follow directions or cautions on a medical alert tag if he has one. If he is conscious he may give you directions. A nitroglycerine tablet may be placed under the tongue or a amyl nitrate ampul broken and held under the nose.

Abdominal Pain

Abdominal pains may be caused by a variety of conditions. Some represent a real emergency. The pain may vary from a dull ache to a sharp stabbing pain. Some are constant and some are intermittent. It may be just an ordinary "belly-ache" from eating too much of the wrong kind of food. If it persists or is accompanied by nausea, vomiting, diarrhea, or constipation, one should not wait to contact a doctor or take home remedies.

Appendicitis

Appendicitis is the most important common illness associated with abdominal pain. It may be indicated by a pain in the pit of the stomach, nausea, and a diarrhea-like feeling. The pain shifts to the right lower side of the abdomen, which becomes tender to touch. Fever may appear, around 99 to 102 degrees F. The symptom of pain is deceptive in that it may move almost anywhere in the abdomen.

Never give anyone who possibly has appendicitis anything to eat or drink, or a laxative, or any other medication. The patient should be placed in a semi-reclining position with a pillow under his knees and an ice bag wrapped in a towel applied to the lower right of the abdomen. While heat may be helpful for some abdominal and back pains, it should not be used if there is a possibility that the condition is appendicitis. The patient should be seen by a doctor as soon as possible.

Gallstones

A person with a history of gall bladder trouble (stomach distress, gas, belching) may have gallstones. The pain characteristically starts in the upper right side and radiates to the right shoulder or to the back, causing the person to double up in cramp-like agony. Repetitive vomiting may occur, eventually producing green bile.

Care by a physician is necessary. The patient should be placed in a semi-reclining position. Heat from a hot water bag or electrical hot pad may be helpful. The doctor will give sedation for the severe pain.

Ulcers

Heartburn or a boring pain in the stomach area which occurs more frequently than once a week could be the first symptom of an ulcer. An antacid preparation may relieve pain. Aspirin should not be taken. The person should be under the care of a physician.

A perforated ulcer produces severe abdominal pain, severe prostration, and shock. The abdominal muscles are very rigid. There is vomiting and a subnormal temperature. The person is in grave danger. Get the victim to the hospital immediately. Notify the doctor in advance so that the operating room will be ready.

Food Poisoning

Abdominal pain, cramps, nausea, vomiting, and diarrhea are signs of food poisoning. Contact with a doctor is necessary to order lab tests to identify the specific type of poisoning and to prescribe medication. Antibiotics can be given to combat the organism. Paregoric can relieve the cramping. Treatment includes correcting the dehydration which occurs as a result of the vomiting and diarrhea. Care must be taken to prevent recontamination.

Hernia

The occurrence of a hernia or rupture rarely takes place suddenly, but occasionally a hernia in the groin will become painful and swollen rapidly. If it cannot be pushed back into the abdominal cavity, strangulation or blockage of circulation to that tissue may occur, causing possible gangrene and a blocked intestine. The patient should get to bed and lie flat on his back. Someone else should elevate the foot of the bed a few inches. Gentle manipulation of the hernia may help it go back. If this doesn't work, apply an ice bag to the hernia to reduce the tenderness and size. After about a half hour repeat the manipulation. In the meantime contact the doctor and follow his instructions. Any suspected hernia or persistent or recurrent pain in the groin should be reported to the doctor.

Nausea and Vomiting

Nausea is sickness in the stomach. A chain of waves pass through the walls of the stomach moving upward rather than downward as usual. There is a forewarning urge to vomit. Vomiting is a powerful contraction of the stomach and diaphram, throwing the contents of the stomach through the esophagus and out of the mouth and sometimes through the nose. While nausea is not a disease, it is a symptom of many diseases ranging from mild maladies to severe emergencies. If vomiting persists or contains blood, a doctor should be contacted immediately.

Diarrhea

Diarrhea accompanies many conditions and treatment rests with the correction of the condition. Medical help may be necessary to do this. Commercial preparations for diarrhea may help, but they should be taken according to your doctor's advice. Other than this, the person should take nothing by mouth for up to twelve hours. Chew on crushed ice to allay thirst. Later sips of water, ginger ale, tea, Seven-Up, or clear broth should be taken at frequent intervals. Stay on these liquids for another twenty-four hours. In the meantime get plenty of bed rest. If there are abdominal cramps, an electric heating pad or hot water bottle may help. After the diarrhea is stopped the person can gradually start to eat light bland foods. Raw fruits and vegetables, spicy foods, rich and fatty foods are to be avoided.

Constipation

Constipation is a frequent cause of abdominal and back pains. It is the retention of solid waste material within the bowel for an unusually long time, or undue difficulty in its evacuation. Habitual failure to respond to the body's signals, a diet lacking in bulk foods or liquids, inactivity, or irregular digestive processes may lead to constipation. A rectal suppository or an enema (3 oz. of mineral or olive oil at bath temperature) will probably provide relief. If not, call your doctor. You should get your doctor's advice for avoiding the condition in the future.

Urinary Retention

Acute inability to urinate and urinary retention is distressing and painful. It may be due to infection, blood clots, bladder stones, enlarged prostate gland, or inactivity. The patient should take a warm bath or apply warm moist packs to the lower abdominal and genital area. If the patient cannot void within an hour, call your doctor. This condition or painful urination should be reported to the doctor.

Back Pains

Kidney Stones

A very excruciating pain, which may start in the back above the waist on either side and may travel down the side of the abdomen into the groin and genital area, may be caused by kidney stones. Nausea and vomiting and frequent desire to urinate may also be present. Urination may cause a burning and an occasional passage of blood in the urine. This condition may be caused by stones in the kidney or ureter. A doctor should be contacted. The patient will get some relief from a hot bath followed by the application of heat to the painful area. All urine should be saved in a clean glass container so the doctor can examine it.

Low Back Pain

Acute backache may be due to muscle strain. Pain may start at the time of injury or later when a muscle spasm catches the victim. He may be unable to move without assistance. It may be a "slipped disc." A doctor's examination will be necessary to determine the cause. The patient may be more comfortable if he will lie down on a flat, hard surface with the knees bent. An electric heating pad may be placed under the area of discomfort. Gentle massage may help, but it should *not* be done directly over the affected muscles. After the spasms have come under control, supportive strappings may be applied to the back by a doctor or other qualified individual.

Other Back Pains

A "slipped disc," arthritis of the spine, constipation, poor posture, or a spastic colon may also cause back pain. A doctor's examination is necessary to determine the cause.

Cramps

Dysmenorrhea

Painful menstruation may be due to an organic condition such as inflammation, a turned uterus, or endocrine disturbance. If so, only competent medical care will bring relief. Reports indicate that occasionally menstrual disturbances are due to allergic factors. More often general health measures and exercise will improve the physical and emotional well-being and diminish the problems at the time of the period. Mild sedatives, applications of heat, and plenty of rest will help relieve the discomfort.

Cramps

Cramps can be very painful. They may affect muscles anywhere in the body, or may occur in the intestines, gallbladder, or uterus. They occur primarily in the calves and feet. They may occur during exercise, stretching, or rest. A cramp occurs when a muscle contracts and will not relax again. Gently massaging the affected muscle or working the limb will relax the muscle and relieve the painful contraction. Heat application will also help. If cramps re-occur frequently (several times a month) consult a physician so that the underlying cause can be found and appropriate treatment administered.

Growing Pains

So-called "growing pains" should always arouse suspicion of something wrong, for normal growing is painless. Chest pains may be due to overexertion, injury, pleurisy, rheumatic fever, or some other heart or lung disease. Joint pain may indicate the beginning of arthritis or rheumatic fever. Painful feet may indicate arthritis, gout, poor circulation, diabetes, corns or calluses, poor-fitting shoes or hose, overweight, overexertion, or too much standing. Treating the symptoms may help, but any of these conditions may require medical attention to determine the cause and to prescribe the treatment.

Skeletal Injuries

Sprains and Strains

There is generally pain associated with skeletal injuries. Sometimes the pain is present at first and other times the pain occurs later. If there is a possibility that the injury involves a fracture or dislocation, it should be treated as a fracture. It should be immobilized and medical help should be secured. Soft tissue injury surrounding the fracture, sore joints, sprains, strains, and bruises can be helped by cold applications. Cold minimizes the swelling and thus reduces the pain and hastens the recovery. If possible place the injured limb in cold tap water or ice water for thirty minutes every two hours for eight hours. If you cannot do this, you may use an ice pack or compress. If an ice cap or ice bag is used, fill it about half full of finely chopped ice, expel the air, and apply it to the contour of the injured limb. An ice compress is made by spreading out a towel and covering half of it, except at the borders, with an inch layer of crushed ice. Fold the other half and the borders over so the ice will not spill. Before applying the ice pack, first cover the injured area with flannel. Leave the cold application in place for thirty minutes, no longer. Remove the pack, dry the area, and cover the part with dry flannel. Repeat the application every two hours for eight hours. Throughout the process, observe the skin to avoid reactions to the cold. Do not let the skin warm up too quickly. In the meantime, elevate the injured area and allow it to rest. After twenty-four hours, apply heat packs to encourage circulation and reduction in swelling.

Bursitis

The bursa is a smooth fibrous sack filled with fluids which provides frictionless movement of tendons as they slide over bones and joints. Injury or irritation resulting in inflammation of these tissues is bursitis. With bursitis certain movements are very painful. Complete rest of the part and application of heat are often helpful. Some medications are helpful in relieving the inflammation. Sometimes fluid can be drawn from the sack with a hypodermic needle. Sometimes operations are necessary.

Types of Unconsciousness

Unconsciousness can be caused by anything which disturbs or impairs the function of the brain. It can range from fainting, which is usually harmless, to deep coma that is near unto death. Also there is the semi-conscious condition in which the victim seems dazed and confused.

The general approach to unconsciousness includes the following measures in this order. If there is no pulse, the victim needs external cardiac massage. If there is no breathing, first clear the airway and then if necessary start artificial respiration. Then control bleeding and treat for shock. Next, call the doctor. The doctor may request the vital signs — temperature, pulse, respiration (TPR).

Examine the victim and the surroundings carefully. They may give a clue to the cause of the unconsciousness. Electric wires, poison containers, evidence of injury to the head, odor on the breath, size of the pupils, blood-tinged saliva, and a medical identification card may help.

Place the victim so that any blood, vomitus, or other fluids can easily flow from his mouth and so that his tongue will stay forward and leave the air passage open. Keep the victim comfortable and warm. Do not move him unnecessarily. Note the color of the victim's face. Its hue (one of the colors of the U.S. flag) can suggest the cause of the unconsciousness, what to look for, and what to do until medical help arrives.

Red Unconsciousness

Increased pressure within the skull results in congestion of blood vessels of the face so that it appears red or flushed. This may result from a stroke or skull injuries. Lay the person down, but raise his head slightly. Give nothing by mouth. Apply cold packs to the head. Use covers to keep him warm, move only when necessary and then by stretcher, and call a doctor.

White Unconsciousness

A drop in blood pressure has resulted from shock or hemorrhage. Lay the person down with the feet and hips elevated. If he is conscious give him a half glass of water unless he is nauseated. Cover the patient with blankets to keep him warm. Move only when necessary and then by stretcher. Call the doctor.

Blue Unconsciousness

An inadequate supply of oxygen in the blood suggests asphyxiation. There will be a weak pulse and absent or irregular breathing. Remove the cause of the asphyxiation — such as remove the victim from a gas-filled room, removing source of electrocution, etc. Lay the person down. Start artificial respiration immediately if breathing is absent. Keep the victim warm.

Causes of Unconsciousness

Fainting

If a person feels faint he should lie flat on the floor and lift his legs straight up. Next best, if he is unable or unwilling to do this, is to sit with his legs wide apart and put his head between them, or to stand with his legs apart and bend forward at the waist so that his head is about at the level of his knees. It is much better to lie down than to receive an injury from falling down.

If a person faints he will usually regain consciousness after his body falls into a horizontal position and blood flow returns to the brain. He should be placed flat. His legs may be elevated. Loosen any tight clothing around the neck. Provide fresh air if possible. If a blanket is available, use it to help keep him warm. Protection from the cold floor is as important as cover. After he has regained consciousness, encourage him to stay on his back for ten minutes or until he feels well enough to sit up. Let him remain sitting up for awhile — ten to fifteen minutes. Then assist him up and let him walk around if he feels well enough. Although simple fainting usually is no real emergency, its occurrence should be reported to your doctor at your earliest convenience so that he can record it in your medical record. However, if unconsciousness lasts for more than five minutes, if fainting recurs, or if faintness persists, you should call the doctor immediately.

Concussion

A severe blow to the head may cause unconsciousness. In some cases a person who appears to be unharmed immediately after an accident will develop problems hours or days afterwards. Have him lie down and keep him quiet. If he is unconscious, turn him on his side. If his face is red, place a pillow under his head. If his face is pale, do not use a pillow but keep his head level with the rest of his body. Keep him comfortable and warm. Do not give him anything to eat or drink. If there is an open wound, gently dress and bandage the wound, but if there is a depression in the skull do not apply pressure. If the victim must be moved, keep him in a horizontal position and avoid jostling him. If a victim has been unconscious, even for a few seconds, he is considered to have suffered a concussion — temporary interruption of brain activity. There may be a headache and nausea. The doctor may call for bed rest for twenty-four hours or longer. After the person has returned to normal activities he should be watched for delayed reaction such as persistent or frequent headaches, inability to concentrate and forgetfulness, vision problems, nausea, drowsiness, dizziness, irritability, or marked changes in normal behavior patterns. If these occur, the person should receive medical attention.

Stroke

Symptoms of stroke vary markedly. They may include headache, weakness, or paralysis of one or more limbs or parts of the body; difficulty in speaking, drooping of one side of the face, nausea, vomiting, dizziness, drowsiness, unconsciousness, or deep coma. The face may be red and veins in the neck standing out. There would be a strong pulse. Breathing may be noisy. Pupils may be of unequal size.

Call for the physician. Lay the patient down, but raise his head slightly. He should be turned on his side so he won't choke on his vomitus or droolings from his mouth. Do not attempt to give fluids or medicine. If breathing has stopped, give mouth-to-mouth or artificial respiration. Apply cold packs to the head. Use covers to keep him warm. Move only when necessary and then use a stretcher.

Drugs

Alcohol, drugs, or other forms of poisoning can cause unconsciousness. The mere presence of alcohol on the breath should not lead a person to disregard other causes of unconsciousness. The person may have been drinking, but some other emergency may have caused his stupor or unconsciousness.

Other Causes of Unconsciousness

Other kinds of accidental injury may also cause unconsciousness, such as electrical shock and gas poisoning. The victim of gas poisoning should be removed from the gas environment. The source of electrical shock should be safely removed before other aid is given. Artificial respiration may be necessary. Other medical conditions already mentioned in this chapter can cause unconsciousness. They include asthmatic attacks, choking, heart attacks, and severe pain. The three remaining topics — convulsions, diabetic emergencies, and heat reactions will also cause unconsciousness.

Convulsions

Convulsions are an attack of unconsciousness accompanied by severe involuntary contractions of the muscles, resulting from a disorder in the nerves controlling the muscles. They may result from certain poisonings, infection, fever, or some injury to the nervous system. Most frequently convulsions occur among children, except for epileptic convulsions which are somewhat different.

Childhood Convulsions

While convulsions are alarming to watch, death rarely occurs from the convulsion itself. Nevertheless, they should never be ignored. A medical investigation to find the cause and prevention should take place, so call a physician at once.

The contractions may start with twitching in a small part of the body such as the face, above the eyes. Then the contractions spread to generalized convulsive motions. The body may become stiff and may bow. Put the child on a soft place like a wide bed or rug. Loosen all clothing. During the convulsion breathing may stop momentarily. If it doesn't begin within a minute, start artificial respiration. After a few minutes the convulsion will gradually subside and leave the victim semiconscious or in a deep sleep. He should be laid on his side to prevent him from choking on his tongue or on fluids. Gently put him to bed and keep him warm and quiet.

If the convulsion is due to a high fever, it is desirable to reduce the child's temperature rapidly. Wrap him in lukewarm moist sheets. A fan will aid evaporation and cooling. Cool sponges and a cool enema also help reduce the temperature. Care should be taken not to bring the temperature down far enough to cause chilling.

If a seizure from other causes doesn't subside, warm packs and a warm enema may be given.

Epileptic Seizures

Epileptic seizures may be more severe (grand mal), or they may be mild (petite mal). In the petite mal, they merely stare ahead unaware of anything. In the grand mal, they may throw themselves about. To avoid injury, one should try to move objects they may strike. One should not try to restrain a victim. It may be possible to place a thick wad of cloth or similar material between the patient's teeth to keep him from biting his tongue or breaking his teeth. It may be possible to put some padding between the victim's head and the floor to keep him from injuring his head. But usually it is best to make little of the convulsion and avoid becoming excited.

Most attacks terminate by themselves and the victim may appear confused for a few moments. He may want to rest or he may go directly into a deep sleep. It is best to lie him on his side so breathing won't be hampered by the tongue or aspirated vomitus or other fluids. Keep him warm and allow him to rest. Psychological care after the attack is important, but undue sympathy may embarrass him. Modern medication controls most epileptic conditions very well today. If an attack occurs, it should be reported to the patient's doctor.

Diabetic Emergencies

Two emergencies may occur to a diabetic — diabetic coma or insulin shock. A diabetic under medical care and following a prescribed routine may never experience one of these emergencies, but if his normal routine of eating, activity, and insulin injection is altered, he may.

Diabetic Coma

If there is too little insulin for the amount of sugar in the blood, diabetic coma (acidosis or hypoinsulinism) may occur. The patient may complain of weakness, drowsiness, excessive thirst, and increased urination. The skin is usually dry and flushed. There may be a fever. Breathing is deep and rapid. The pulse is weak and rapid. There is an acetone or sweetish breath. The drowsiness may progress into a coma. The symptoms may come on slowly and the victim may be able to take the necessary action. If not, he may become stuporous and confused. Call his doctor right away and keep the patient warm, quiet, and comfortable. If a doctor cannot be reached, treat for shock. Give fluids not containing sugar or starch. If the victim is unconscious or vomiting, administer fluid (1 teaspoon of salt to 1 quart of water) by rectum.

Insulin Shock

If there is too much insulin for the amount of sugar, a reaction to insulin (alkalosis or hyperinsulinism) may take place. The patient may complain of hunger, sweating, nervousness, dizziness, and headache. The skin is moist and pale, breathing is normal and shallow, pulse is full and strong, confusion may progress to unconsciousness. Convulsions may occur. Immediately give the patient some hard candy, sugar, honey, or a drink containing sugar. If he is unconscious, put the candy under the tongue. Then call the doctor and keep the patient quiet and comfortable.

Heat Reaction

Fever

Fever is a warning signal that trouble is present. It is also an internal defense against disease. Sometimes the body overdoes its defense and the fever becomes dangerous, and steps must be taken to reduce it. Children tend to react with higher temperatures than adults. Temperatures of 105 degrees and above can be hazardous. When a temperature approaches 104 degrees, put the patient to bed and call a doctor. If the doctor cannot be reached, try to lower the temperature by giving aspirin and giving a sponge bath. Sponge a portion of the body at a time keeping the rest of the body covered, administer a tepid or lukewarm enema. Apply an ice bag or cold cloths to the head. If conscious, give water or ice chips by mouth. Keep track of the temperature so that these measures can be stopped when the temperature is reduced to a safe point.

Heatstroke

Exposure to heat or direct sun can result in heatstroke or sunstroke. It results from failure of the body to lower its own temperature. Sweating ceases and the body's temperature rises excessively. This high fever can cause permanent damage to organs such as the brain, kidneys, or liver. Convulsions may occur. It is dangerous unless treated promptly. Usually the victim is observed after he has collapsed. His skin is flushed, very dry, and very hot. Medical help is needed. Treatment can begin immediately. Remove him to a cool place. Cool the body by sponging it, or by placing him in a tub of cold water. Continue until the temperature drops to 102 degrees. He will require medical and probably hospital treatment.

Heat Exhaustion

Heat exhaustion is less serious than heatstroke. It is a different reaction to heat and a different treatment is required. It is associated with profuse perspiration. The person becomes fatigued and faint, has white clammy skin, a weak pulse, shallow breathing, and may lose consciousness briefly. It is much like fainting, but hot weather and heavy work suggests heat exhaustion. The victim should lie down with his head lower than his body. Loosen tight clothing. Move him to a cool place, but be careful that he doesn't get chilled. If he is conscious, give him 1/2 glass of cool salt water (1/2 teaspoon salt per 1/2 glass water) every fifteen minutes. Call a doctor. Do not let him sit up for some time. Keep him quiet in a cool place until he feels entirely recovered.

Heat Cramps

Prolonged working in an atmosphere where one sweats excessively and drinks a lot of water may cause heat cramps through loss of body salts. Symptoms include severe muscle cramps, especially in the calf of the leg and in the abdomen, faintness, dizziness, and exhaustion. Treatment and prevention involves getting adequate amounts of salt. The best source is coated salt tablets taken with plenty of water. Severe cases may require medical attention and salt administration intravenously.

Some Nosebleeds Are Serious

Nosebleed from a whack on the nose is disturbing enough, but when blood gushes for no apparent reason, you have a right to be concerned.

Most cases of nosebleed are the logical result of mishap, injury or irritation from colds or allergy, and when bleeding stops in ten minutes or so, there is no cause for alarm. The simplest cases arise from a sneeze, a bump or a scrape and represent ruptures of blood vessels close to the surface of the front part of the nose. If customary remedies fail to stem the flow or if episodes come often, better consult a doctor.

Sudden, frequent or prolonged bleeding from the nose can be a sign of a wide variety of disorders. Unexplained episodes can mean some defect in the blood is interfering with proper clotting. Recurrent nosebleed may accompany such dread blood diseases as hemophilia and leukemia, and it can suggest rheumatic fever. Other symptoms often occur first and nosebleed alone is no reason to panic.

Victims of high blood pressure, especially if they've been under mental or physical stress, occasionally bleed from the back of the nose. Or the bleeding may be due to blood-thinning drugs, in which case the dosage may have to be adjusted. Two unlikely causes of nosebleed are scurvy, which is a serious deficiency of vitamin C, or a tiny tumor inside the nose.

For stubborn cases in which injury or irritation are to blame, the physician may have to resort to cauterization, an essentially painless way of sealing broken vessels with chemicals or an electric needle. Or he may pack the nose with sterile gauze, then apply a natural coagulant to the main area of bleeding. For certain rare clotting disorders, vitamin K is sometimes prescribed.

If you are ever called upon to act in a nosebleed emergency, the first thing to do is try to keep the patient as quiet as possible. Have him sit in a chair with his head tilted forward and blow out the clotted blood. Next, moisten a ball of cotton with nose drops, cold water or peroxide and gently insert it into the bleeding nostril. Then pinch the nostrils together firmly for at least five minutes.

Placing ice on the bridge of the nose or cold compresses on the neck, by the way, probably does more to divert the patient than to stop the nosebleed.

After the bleeding stops, leave the cotton in place for several hours. To keep the clot that has formed intact, caution the patient against blowing his nose.

If after you've done your best and home treatment hasn't been successful, call a doctor promptly. The case obviously calls for stronger measures.

Reprinted with permission from *Changing Times, the Kiplinger Magazine*, December 1971, Vol. 25, No. 12, p. 41. Copyright 1971 by the Kiplinger Washington Editors, Inc., 1729 H. Street NW, Washington, D.C. 20006.

Facts about Electricity

Basic Information About Electricity

What Is Electricity?

Electricity is a form of energy, just as heat, light, and sound are forms of energy. It can neither be created nor destroyed, at least not by ordinary means. Electricity is contained in and derived from all matter that occupies space and has weight. Electricity, then, is present in those things that surround us. All matter contains tiny particles called atoms. Each atom has its own protons, neutrons, and electrons. Protons and neutrons stick close together, whereas electrons can be "moved" quite easily from one atom to another. The movement of electrons from one atom to the next is what we call electricity. . . .

Electricity and You

How Does Shock Occur?

Shock and related injuries may occur when the body becomes a part of this circuit or closed loop. You may become a part of an existing circuit by touching both wires of an energized circuit, or you may create an unintentional circuit back to earth by touching an energized wire or an energized conductive object while your body is directly or indirectly in contact with the earth.

What Determines the Severity of the Shock?

The severity of the shock received as a result of an accidental contact with an electric circuit depends upon a number of factors:

(1) The amount (rate of current flow measured in amperes) and duration (exposure time) of the current flow.

(2) Part of the body through which current flows (current flowing from one finger to another of the same hand would *not* pass through vital organs and, therefore, would not be fatal, although a burn might result).

(3) Resistance offered by the body. As the skin becomes progressively moist, its resistance decreases and will allow more current to pass through it.

(4) Type of circuit with which contact is made. The pulsations of the 60-cycle, 120-volt alternating currents (A.C.) normally found in most homes in the

Reprinted from *Demonstration Guide for Prevention of Electric Shock Injury*, Consumer Protection and Environmental Health Service, Public Health Service Publication No. 1952, pp. 7-9 and 13, Environmental Control Administration, Bureau of Community Environmental Management, United States Department of Health, Education and Welfare, 1969.

United States are more pronounced in producing a physiological response than are equivalent uninterrupted direct (D.C.) currents.

Also, at much higher frequencies than experienced in the home (above 60 cycles) the body does not experience any sensation to current flow except heat. One of the present-day medical uses of electricity in which this principle is applied is in diathermy apparatus.

(5) Other factors that may affect the degree of shock include:

    (a) Phase of the heart cycle when shock occurs (applies to momentary contact);

    (b) Age, size, and physical condition of person.

What Are the Physiological Effects of Varying Amounts of Current Flow?

The physiological effects of electric shock result from passage of the electric current through the body. There are no precise limits which determine the exact injury from any given amount of current flow (measured in amperes). The following chart, however, gives approximate measurements of injury related to amperage:

Amount of current, in milliamperes* (1 ampere = 1,000 milliamperes)	=	Fraction of total potential current flow from a typical 15-ampere wall outlet	=	Physiological response
Less than 1/2		1/30,000		No sensation
1/2 to 2		1/30,000-1/7,500		Threshold of perception
2 to 10		1/7,500-1/1,500		Muscular contraction (mild to strong)
5 to 25		1/3,000-1/600		Painful shock, inability to let go
Over 25		1/600		Violent muscular contraction
50 to 200		1/300-1/75		Heart convulsions, death (fibrillation)
Over 100		1/150		Paralysis of breathing, burns

*For comparison, a 100-watt light bulb consumes about 1,000 milliamperes.

What Is Voltage and its Relationship to the Shock Hazard?

Voltage is the difference in electrical pressure between two substances and/or objects. Earth is considered as having zero voltage.

Voltage is what provides electricity with the ability to overcome the resistance presented by materials and substances through which electricity may tend to flow. Resistance to current flow varies greatly from item to item and is measured in ohms.

Because of varying physiological makeup of the body, it is difficult to establish a definite voltage sufficient to overcome man's natural skin resistance to the extent that a shock hazard exists. A value of 30 volts *alternating current*, however, has received wide acceptance for indoor application (outdoor application may be as low as 12 volts). When the voltage is increased to the 120-240 volts used in most homes, a definite shock hazard exists. . . .

Removal and Emergency Care of Victim

Breaking contact with the electrical circuit should be done as promptly as possible. A dry stick, dry rope, dry coat, newspaper, or other dry nonconductor may be used to free the victim where immediate de-energizing of the conductor is not possible.

Mouth-to-mouth artificial respiration is a great life-saving measure in electric shock, gas poisoning, drowning, and in other emergencies that result in the cessation of breathing. To be effective, it must be applied immediately after rescue and should be continued until normal breathing has been restored, or until death is certain.

The unconscious person often needs to be protected from further strain on his vitality, which already is weakened. As far as possible, keep him covered and warm both during and after resuscitation. Do not permit the patient to exert himself. If it should be necessary to move him, keep him lying down.

Never give liquids to an unconscious person. They may choke him. To avoid strain on the heart, when the victim revives, he should be kept lying down and not allowed to stand or sit. Seek medical assistance as soon as possible.

First Aid for Common Sports Injuries

In Diving Injuries . . . Splint 'Em Where They Float'

One July day, an 11-year-old girl dived into an above-the-ground swimming pool in her back yard and, instead of coming right to the surface, began sinking to the bottom. Her companions immediately jumped in and pulled her out of the water by her hair and lowered her the four feet to the ground. Today, the girl is a quadriplegic.

A 20-year-old man, about to be married, dived into a pool and hit one of the sloping sides. It was obvious that he was injured. His companions leaped to his assistance. But instead of pulling him out of the pool, they supported him in the water until help arrived. While still in the water, the young man was placed on a spine board. A few weeks after the accident, he walked down the aisle with his bride.

The difference in the outcome of these two cases — in which each patient had a severe cervical fracture — was in the immediate handling. But according to surgeon Richard W. Rado of Riverdale, N.J., too few victims of diving mishaps get the kind of treatment the young man received.

For more than six years, he has been campaigning to educate his colleagues, first-aid squads, lifeguards, and the general public on the proper handling of watersport injuries. A film he made on the subject, "Safe Handling of Diving Injuries," has won a National Safety Foundation certificate of merit.

Dr. Rado notes that doctors have been increasingly successful in making the general public aware of the dangers of moving acutely injured patients. "It would be rare indeed at the scene of an auto accident not to hear someone in the crowd say, 'Don't move the patient.' It is to the credit of the medical profession that the basic principle of 'splint 'em where they lie' has been so widely disseminated to the lay public and accepted."

The exact converse, Dr. Rado complains, seems to be the rule in water or diving accidents. Since drowning is the danger uppermost in the layman's mind, Dr. Rado understands the priority given to getting the injured person out of the water. "However, in this type of injury, the basic principle of not moving the patient probably obtains to an even greater degree than in automobile and other accidents." He adds that cervical spine injury is more prone to result in cord transection than any other vertebral fracture.

"Little imagination is required to visualize a patient being pulled into a boat by traction in the armpits while someone is also pushing him from below," Dr. Rado comments. "The flailing neck of the child whose father carries him from the water with one arm under the back and the other under the thighs needs no

Reprinted with permission from *Emergency Medicine,* July 1969.

further description. It seems inconceivable that anyone could be removed from an above-the-ground pool, carried over its edge, then lowered four feet, without further injury to an already broken neck — unless a rigid spine support is used. Yet cases of each of these types of removal occur."

Dr. Rado's special interest in these injuries was aroused 15 years ago, when he was an intern on ambulance duty at Newark City Hospital. One afternoon the ambulance was summoned to a public swimming pool where a boy had been injured.

"When I got there, a 17-year-old boy had been lugged to a field house 50 feet from the pool," Dr. Rado recalls. "Totally paralyzed, the boy was lying on a sagging iron bedstead. The poor kid had been hauled out of the water, carried without a stretcher, and dropped on the bed. It was obvious that he had a broken neck and should not have been moved without a rigid spine board under him."

Soon after Dr. Rado opened his practice in the lake region of northern New Jersey, he saw a number of similarly mishandled persons with cervical or other spinal fractures sustained in the water. In the case of the little girl who was permanently paralyzed after suffering such an injury, Dr. Rado feels the outcome might have been much different if she had been left in the water until a support could have been placed under her head and back.

"The 20-year-old fellow who was handled properly had the worst cervical fracture the orthopedist said he had ever seen," notes Dr. Rado. "The patient had to undergo an open reduction at C-5 and C-6 and then Crutchfield tongs were inserted. Yet he was out of the hospital in three weeks with no neurological deficit.

"Unfortunately," says Dr. Rado, "people panic when there is a water accident. When the water is very rough or extremely cold or when there is excessive bleeding, it may make it impossible to keep a person in the water. But in the majority of cases, it is better to do so."

Dr. Rado believes that keeping the patient afloat until trained help arrives with a spine board "has much to commend it. The water makes a fine support, and the patient can be easily maintained afloat with minimal hand support and with the neck in neutral position. Application of the spine board is then accomplished by sliding it under him and letting it float up.

"An airway must, of course, be established if the patient is having trouble breathing. But even mouth-to-mouth resuscitation may be done in the water.

"A rigid support should be placed under the victim in the water as soon as possible. The support may be a spine board, a surf board, an aquaplane, a wooden plank, a water ski, a door, an ironing board, or even a picnic bench. Don't select anything that may break or bend, such as a Styrofoam paddleboard, sailing board, or inflated mattress.

"If you have a choice," Dr. Rado emphasizes, "bring the support to the victim, not the victim to the support. In rough water or in water beyond the surf breakers, it is preferable to support, move, or float the victim in a position parallel to the waves and swells. Get the rigid support under the victim and tie him on before coming ashore through the surf. A large beach towel, several regular towels tied together, bathrobe ties, or rope may be used to encircle the support and the victim's body. If only one tie is available, encircle the chest area."

Dr. Rado says there are more neck and spine injuries in water accidents than are reported. He notes that in one recent week, at the 120-bed Chilton Memorial Hospital in Pompton Plains, where he is a staff surgeon, three patients were admitted with broken necks sustained in water accidents. An investigation of the cases showed that the patients were removed from the water with "little thought to the possibility of other injuries."

According to Dr. Rado, at least 500 persons become quadriplegic each year from water accidents in the United States, five times the number caused by polio. He says the leading cause of such injuries is diving from a board or other elevation. Next are diving into waves and diving into shallow water.

"Every beach should be required to have a spine board available for such emergencies," says Dr. Rado. "The injured person should be placed on the board and wet towels rolled and placed on each side of the head to keep the victim from moving his neck. The patient should be taken to the hospital without being moved from the board. And in the emergency room, X-rays should be taken with the patient still on the board.

"Because of the growth of backyard and other private pools, it is vital that doctors inform everyone they can about how important it is to handle victims of water accidents properly. We can't expect laymen to become diagnosticians, but the use of water spine boards for *any* accident should be a must. After all, the patients who might benefit the most from correct treatment may very easily be the ones in whom the nature of the injury isn't evident," says Dr. Rado. "Perhaps 'splint 'em where they float' should be the water safety equivalent of the now generally accepted 'splint 'em where they lie.' "

Cryokinetics

James P. Juvenal

Ice has been used as an immediate therapeutic agent for many years, principally for arresting and reducing swelling. That it effectively does this, everyone agrees. The problem lies in the duration of the application.

Since there's no accurate way to determine just how much soft-tissue damage or vascular involvement has occurred in a specific injury, the coach or trainer can only make an educated guess on how long to maintain the coldness and immobilization. The period may vary anywhere from one to 48 hours.

Once the swelling has been reduced, heat and mild exercise are prescribed. The heat increases circulation, thus producing a more rapid absorption of the exudate. If, however, the exudate has congealed during the immobilization period, it's possible that the heat will *increase* the swelling and thus *prolong* the recovery time.

On the other hand, a careful movement of the injured area can prove beneficial. The forceful "milking" of the involved tissues and vessels can reduce the hematoma and thus reduce the recovery time.

Two factors militate against such movement: (1) the possibility of further injury and trauma, and (2) the severe pain usually caused by forceful movement. These two factors were kept in mind in the development of a new therapeutic concept known as cryokinetics (*cryo*-cold, *kinetics*-movement).

It was discovered that a *mild* local anesthetic could provide sufficient freedom from pain to allow forceful motion. The word "mild" is important. If sensation were completely eliminated — through the use of novocaine, for example — more extensive damage could result.

Hence, a mild anesthetic that reduces pain to a tolerable minimum must be used. This "tolerable pain" relieves the subject without covering up any symptoms of further injury resulting from vigorous movement. Ice represents an excellent anesthetic for this purpose.

A pioneer in the application of cryokinetics for orthopedic injuries is Dr. Ernst Dehne, former Chief of Orthopedics, Brooke Army Medical Center, San Antonio, Tex. He believes that ice is not only beneficial in the immediate treatment of traumatic orthopedic injuries but is an effective rehabilitative agent as well. He applies cryokinetic techniques to sprains (ligament tears) of the foot and ankle, contusions, localized burns, and minor fractures.

Basically, the application of cryokinetics is quite simple. The injury is first thoroughly examined to eliminate the possibility of fracture. Ice is then applied, either by ice-water immersion or ice massage, depending on the injury's location.

Reprinted with permission from *Scholastic Coach*, September 1969.

Once the area is adequately anesthetized, exercise is begun. When pain returns (thawing), the procedure is repeated. Several repetitions are made each day until the athlete returns to competition.

At Robert E. Lee H.S. we had some definite apprehensions about adopting this seemingly "radical" method. But after discussions with Dr. Dehne and several team physicians, we decided to use it in our training room.

In cryokinetics, ice is used in three forms:

1. Ice-water immersion — on ankles, hands, and feet. The injured part is immersed in water at room temperature. Ice is then gradually added.

2. Crushed ice — generally used at the field. The injured part is packed in crushed ice and wrapped securely in a damp towel.

3. Ice massage — on body areas not easily immersed. Water is frozen in a clean tin can (soup or juice size), and a tongue depressor is placed in the can so the patient can hold the ice cylinder without freezing his fingers. Water, poured over the can, can easily remove the ice.

During the application, pain is the first sensation experienced. A warming is then felt, and then a degree of numbness. When numbness sets in, forceful exercise is begun and is continued until the pain returns. The procedure is then repeated.

A thorough examination of the injured area must be performed before the cryokinetic treatment is initiated. *If there's any doubt, the area is packed in ice, splinted with a pneumatic splint, and the patient is referred to the team physician.* While it's possible for a trainer or coach to miss on a diagnosis, especially with ankle injuries, this has never happened in our training room.

Exercises used in the cryokinetic treatment aim at a full range of motion and the normal use of the injured parts. Continued ice applications and exercise lend to the rapid achievement of these goals. The injuries are usually strapped after each complete treatment and the patient is given instructions to "use the part as normally as possible." The treatments are repeated several times daily until the patient can compete with minimum pain.

Here are several examples, showing the value of the cryokinetic method:

Moderate Strain of the Quadriceps — examination disclosed pain on knee extension and lateral rotation. Ice massage was applied within five minutes after injury, and the entire area was numbed sufficiently (in five minutes) to begin exercise. The patient suffered no pain on active knee extension and active hip flexion.

He was then instructed to walk around the training room until the pain returned (about three minutes). Ice massage was again applied, and after two minutes the area was again numbed. The patient was then instructed to jog the length of the basketball court until pain returned. After he jogged four lengths, pain returned, and the massage was applied for the third time.

He was then told to sprint the length of the court. He sprinted the distance four times before pain returned. The injured area was then securely wrapped for support. The patient was given two ice cylinders and was instructed to repeat the "freeze-sprint" procedure before retiring and after awakening.

The following morning the patient complained of little pain, but the ice massage procedure was repeated twice. The leg was again wrapped for support and the patient worked out in shorts with the team. After school, he resumed contact work with the leg wrapped in an elastic bandage. In short, he was able to return to full contact work with a minimum of pain in less than 24 hours! Normally this injury would have sidelined the athlete for 48-72 hours, or more.

Severe Medial Sprain of the Left Ankle — patient was in extreme pain and had no mobility in the joint; palpatation showed pain above the medial malleolus, but there was little swelling. The injury was immediately packed in crushed ice, wrapped in a damp towel and splinted. The athlete was transferred to the hospital where X-rays proved negative. The hospital prescribed an elastic wrap and crutches and cold packs for 24 hours (to minimize swelling), and instructed the athlete to stay off the ankle.

After consultation with the team doctor, the athlete, and his parents, we obtained permission to apply the cryokinetic treatment. The treatment was started the following morning with ice-water immersions. After the part was sufficiently anesthetized, we had the athlete begin active exercise, including dorsiflexion, plantar-flexion, and rotation. The patient complained of only minimal pain. After the second immersion, he was instructed to walk around the training room without limping. This was also done with minimum pain.

The ankle was then taped securely and the patient was instructed to keep his foot elevated in class and to actively move the ankle as much as possible. During the noon recess, the patient again repeated the immersion-exercise routine. He was retaped and sent back to class with the same instructions.

The patient was always encouraged to walk as normally as possible. During the afternoon practice, immersion was repeated, and the patient began walking immediately after the first immersion. After the second immersion, the patient was able to jog the length of the court twice with a minimum of pain.

Four subsequent immersions permitted the patient to alternately sprint and jog the length of the court four times with little or no pain. After the fourth immersion, the patient was retaped and instructed to repeat the immersion-jog-sprint procedure twice at home.

The treatment was repeated the next morning, and the athlete sprinted the length of the court several times with little pain. He was taped again and allowed to work out in shorts with the team. On the third day, the immersions were stopped and he resumed full activity with a protective and supportive strapping.

In less than 72 hours, this patient was able to return to full contact with no limitation of movement and a minimum of pain. Normally he'd have been sidelined for two to three weeks.

Lateral Sprain of the Right Ankle – examination revealed severe swelling above and below the lateral malleolus. Further examination ruled out the possibility of fracture, and treatment was begun less than five minutes after injury.

The first immersion brought immediate relief and full motion. The second immersion allowed the patient to walk with *no* pain. The third immersion enabled him to sprint the length of the court four times. The final immersion allowed him to move freely with little pain. The ankle was taped securely and the patient returned to practice *less than one hour* after the sprain.

The injury normally would have kept him out for a week or more. Thanks to the treatment, he played in two basketball games the following day with just minimum pain.

Purpose of Treatment

The adoption of cryokinetics as a standard treatment was prompted by the desire to give each athlete the best possible care under the safest possible conditions, and to allow the athlete to return to action as soon as possible.

The results have been remarkable. The treatment has effected a considerable savings in time, effort, and expense in the care of injuries. Though the exact recovery time varies for each injury, the estimate given in the aforementioned cases are fairly accurate.

The psychological benefits of the treatment are also worthy of mention. Psychological management begins with the initial examination. In the sprained-ankle case, for example, the patient was first instructed to move his toes. This showed him that all of the functions were not lost. The non-affected parts were then palpated to demonstrate that the entire foot wasn't damaged. The patient was further reassured by moving his foot and ankle (which he could do to some extent).

When ice was applied, the pain was so rapidly relieved and the motion so readily attained that the patient was quite gratified. His own participation in the treatment further aided in the psychological adjustment. (Patients should be strongly encouraged to treat themselves – after receiving proper instruction – both at home and in the training room.)

Continued use of cryokinetic treatment will lead to minor changes in its application, but the basic concept of cold-movement should not change. "Charley horse," "wry-neck," and mild hamstring pulls are other injuries that have been successfully treated with cryokinetics. Cryokinetics are also being used to help relieve chronic low back pain, but the results of this venture have not yet been determined.

Cryokinetics has come up with a new answer to that sticky question – "When do you replace cold with heat?" With cryokinetics . . . you don't!

Cold Treatment of Ankle Sprains

Gordon Stoddard

The accepted procedure in treating ankle sprains is to apply ice, compression, and elevation, and follow up with various heat modalities after a 24 to 48 hour period.

No one can really quarrel with this treatment. But we believe we have improved upon it. We've found that the extended use of cold is most beneficial in returning the athlete to competition and eliminating as quickly as possible many of the complicating recovery obstacles, such as swelling, limited function, and pain.

After the injured ankle has been examined, treated initially, X-rayed, and the possibility of fracture or complete ligamentous rupture ruled out, we initiate a five phase program.

Instead of using heat on the subsequent days, we utilize ice immersion followed by therapeutic exercises. Two or three treatments per day are administered in an attempt to reduce swelling, regain the normal range of motion and function, and eliminate pain.

The immersion technique represents the best method of cold application. It produces a dry cold that is more evenly distributed throughout the ankle joint and virtually eliminates pain, allowing for the introduction of exercise and the return of function.

The athlete is fitted with a rubberized boot and his foot and ankle are immersed in an ice slush solution for eight to 12 minutes. The rubberized boot minimizes discomfort and keeps the toes from coming into direct contact with the ice solution.

After complete analgesia or numbness is attained, the exercise phase is initiated. The athlete, after removing the boot, is instructed to exercise the injured ankle passively through the range of motion of the foot and ankle, up to a bearable amount of pain.

Three sets of five repetitions are used in each of the basic movements of plantar flexion, dorsal flexion, inversion, and eversion. The number of repetitions and sets used in each phase is relatively the same.

The second phase of the treatment consists of offering slight resistance to the foot and ankle throughout the basic movements, using pain and the athlete's tolerance as a guideline. As function and strength begin to return, more resistance can be applied in subsequent treatments.

The third phase of treatment and exercise includes isometric contractions throughout the range of joint motion. Resistance is applied for six to eight

Reprinted with permission from *Scholastic Coach,* May 1966.

seconds to assure the maximum contraction of the muscles involved in the basic movements. It's important to offer isometric resistance in more than one angle for each movement.

The fourth phase consists of isotonic exercise based upon the progressive resistance principle.

The final phase of treatment and rehabilitation, initiated after the isotonic exercises have been completed, includes the return of the athlete to active exercise. The basic progression of walking, jogging, running and cutting is followed, emphasizing the use of a normal gait; we don't want the athlete favoring the ankle or substituting other muscle groups by way of compensation.

After the swelling has subsided, the function has returned, and the joint is relatively free of pain, heat is generally used as both a therapeutic agent and a psychological lift. To facilitate the healing process, we employ a limited degree of pulsating ultrasound at low intensity in water, in addition to the whirlpool bath at 100 degrees.

The ice immersion method followed by a progressive exercise program has proved extremely helpful in assuring a safe and early return of the athlete to competition.

When returning the athlete to competition, however, it's vitally important to continue the rehabilitative exercise and to strap the ankle in order to prevent recurrence of the injury.

Simple Treatment for Simple Muscle Injuries

Samuel Homola

A little knowledge may be a dangerous thing, but more often than not it can prove a boon. This particularly applies to muscle injuries. The athlete who knows something about such injuries may be able to reduce both the chances of disability and the subsequent loss of playing time.

For this reason, coaches should, whenever possible, educate their athletes on the basic methods of tending to muscle injuries.

Let's take a look at some of the more common muscle injuries, the cause and prevention of each, and the treatment of such injuries in general.

Contusions

Contusions are, for the most part, simply bruises. They occur whenever a muscle receives a blow hard enough to rupture tiny blood vessels in its belly, causing intramuscular bleeding and muscle spasm.

Sometimes called charley horses, these injuries are difficult to avoid in contact sports, since there's no way to fully protect vulnerable areas from occasional blows during the constant collision between players. Adequate padding, strict enforcement of the rules, and good sportsmanship are essential to the prevention of an excessive number of injuries.

Unusual fatigue, causing the athlete to lose control and timing, is a frequent cause of injury. For this reason, it's always best to relieve a player, at least temporarily, whenever it becomes apparent that fatigue has overtaken him. With a little rest, the reflexes will become sharper and the athlete will be able to protect himself as well as play a better game.

Simple muscle soreness is, by far, the most common muscular complaint among athletes. It's usually induced by the accumulated waste products in a muscle that has undergone unaccustomed exercise, either in type or in amount.

Whenever muscles have been conditioned for a certain kind of exercise, they're usually able to oxidize or neutralize the lactic acid and other metabolites that result from muscular contraction. If, however, the muscles are required to do a little more than usual, or if the exercise is changed in some way, the irritation resulting from an accumulation of lactic acid causes soreness.

Of course, an athlete's ability to recover from exercise improves with training, since the amount of oxygen, buffers, and other chemical substances in the bloodstream (needed in flushing out and recharging an exercised muscle) increases along with physical fitness.

Reprinted with permission from *Scholastic Coach,* March 1966.

Simple muscle soreness usually becomes apparent the day after the unaccustomed exercise, and is mildly symptomatic for only a day or two.

Obviously, the best way for an athlete to avoid muscle soreness is to be careful not to exceed his usual effort by more than a small amount. His training should be progressive so that he gradually works up to the effort that will be required for all-out participation in the activity.

Anytime an athlete grossly exceeds the effort he's accustomed to making, he'll experience muscle soreness, no matter how well trained he is; and whenever there's a sudden change in the type of exercise, the soreness may be acute. The coach must hence be careful not to endanger a scheduled performance by allowing the athlete to participate in another sport or in unaccustomed exercise a day or two before a game.

In any event, a proper warm-up will help prevent excessive muscle soreness, since the increased blood supply will chemically prepare the muscles to handle the waste products of muscular contraction.

A muscle that's forced into heavy exercise without being warmed up with an increased flow of blood may be loaded down with more waste products than the existing blood flow can carry out; and the more of these products that remain in the muscle, the greater will be the amount of soreness.

In addition, an improperly or inadequately warmed up muscle, in failing to remove its waste products from the very beginning of the exercise, may also fail to replenish its energy stores in keeping pace with starting effort. This will produce premature exhaustion, since an increased flow of blood is necessary in converting lactic acid back to glycogen, the source of muscle energy.

Muscular contraction itself is anaerobic; that is, it doesn't require oxygen for the chemical process that utilizes the glycogen. But a steady and increased supply of oxygen is essential for the recovery of continuously exercised muscles.

A sprinter's heart, for example, must pump up to six gallons of blood per minute to supply the amount of oxygen needed to complete a race. If the athlete warms up properly, he can concentrate enough oxygen in his muscles beforehand to get off to a good start, and he'll be able to prolong his starting effort with a faster recovery for continued and unbroken performance. An adequate warm-up will also cut down on muscle soreness.

Muscle Lameness

Muscle lameness, like muscle soreness, stems from unaccustomed exercise, and may not become apparent until the next day. Unlike the soreness caused by an accumulation of waste products, lameness results from microscopic tears in muscle fibers that have been forced to contract against a heavier load than usual. Because of the injury resulting from such effort, soreness and stiffness in the affected muscles may last for three or four days following the exercise.

Since muscle lameness is caused more by forceful contraction than by repeated contraction, progressive resistance exercise that's designed to duplicate or simulate the movements that might produce lameness should be done in order to prevent such disability. Such exercise should also be made progressively harder over a period of time, so that the actual performance of the sport itself will demand less effort than that made in training.

Exercise with barbells and dumbbells, or resistive exercise with additional weight strapped to the body, offers a good way to build strength for athletic competition.

Pulled Muscle

One of the most incapacitating muscular injuries, of course, is the pulled muscle, or a partial separation or tearing of a muscle, either in the muscle fibers or in the tendons. The symptoms associated with this type of injury are usually immediate, the athlete becoming painfully aware that he has sustained an injury.

Complete disability may or may not occur, depending upon the severity of the injury. If there's a complete separation of the muscle, or if a tendon has torn loose from its attachment site, the muscle may snap apart like a broken rubber band, causing obvious deformity in the injured limb. It'll be obvious from the pain and disability that the services of a physician are immediately needed.

The most common cause of muscle tears is an inadequate warm-up. No athlete should ever make a maximum or high-speed effort without first going through a series of lighter, slower movements that duplicate the effort he's about to make.

Whenever cold muscles are forced to contract suddenly, tears often occur in the relaxed or antagonistic muscle fibers. The reason for this is that a cold muscle can contract faster than it can relax. For example, a baseball player who pitches a fast ball without warming up may tear his biceps muscle, even though it's not actively contracted during the pitch.

It's thus usually best to include a few general warm-up exercises in the pre-game routine in order to make sure *all* of the muscles are warmed up before participation. The increased blood flow in warmed-up muscles will increase the intramuscular temperature and lower the viscosity of the muscle tissue so that it'll "give" more readily in sudden contraction or in sudden movements that lengthen the relaxed fibers.

Whenever simple *soreness* occurs, a little light exercise that stimulates the blood flow in the affected muscles will usually relieve the symptoms by flushing out the accumulated waste products.

In cases of *lameness*, however (characterized by unusually stiff and painful muscles), hot baths, light massage, and rest are indicated the first few days, along with simple muscular contractions to prevent adhesions from forming between the injured muscle fibers. After three or four days, the exercise should be made progressively more vigorous, with normal activity being resumed by the end of the week.

The treatment of a *torn muscle* or a severe *contusion* isn't as simple nor the recovery as rapid. Whenever a muscle injury is severe enough to cause bleeding (black and blue discoloration) or immediate disability, it should usually be treated immediately with rest and a cold pack. If the cold can't be applied continuously, it should be applied for about 30 minutes every two hours for 24 to 36 hours.

The chilling effect of the cold will constrict the capillaries in the injured tissues and reduce the swelling as well as relieve the pain.

Whenever an injury occurs in an extremity, the injured part may be plunged into a pan of cold water. If the injury occurs higher up on the arm or leg, or somewhere else on the body, a cold pack must be used.

Cold Pack

An effective cold pack can be made by filling a rubber or plastic container with crushed ice and then wrapping it in a moist towel.

Ethyl chloride spray, or a chemically treated ice bag that gets cold when broken open, sometimes makes a handy cold application in an emergency. Caution must be exercised in the use of ethyl chloride spray; you must be sure to follow the instructions on the bottle. Excessive spraying with an excessive amount of frost can damage the skin with frostbite.

In most cases, *it's best to wait at least 36 hours before applying heat to an injury*, even where the cold applications are discontinued after 24 hours. Use of heat before all of the bleeding has stopped can cause further bleeding, thus increasing swelling and discoloration. If a hot application causes a throbbing pain in the injured tissues, it's wise to go back to cold packs and wait another day or so before trying heat again.

A hot pack can be made by filling a rubber bottle with hot faucet water and then wrapping it in a piece of flannel that has been wrung out in hot water; or you may apply hot, moist flannel and then keep it hot under the light of a heating lamp or an infrared bulb.

Heat may be applied 20 or 30 minutes several times a day, followed by light muscular contractions (through a full range of joint movements) and massage, so long as these ministrations cause no pain and it's apparent that the swelling has started to subside. Hot applications will dilate the blood vessels, increase the flow of blood, and aid in flushing out the accumulated blood and tissue fluid.

The treatment, whether hot or cold, will be more effective if both the application and the body part are covered with a sheet of insulating plastic or rubber to prevent the circulation of air.

Many trainers apply heat for a couple of hours each morning and then wrap the injured area with an analgesic pack to provide a constant surface heat.

Diathermy, a penetrating shortwave heat, can be used in the training room to heat deep muscles. Ultrasound, which penetrates tissues with high-frequency sound waves, is sometimes used by doctors to heat injured muscles and joints.

Contrast bathing — that is, the alternate use of heat and cold — might be useful in reducing swelling and stiffness after the first three or four days. The dilatation and contraction of the small capillaries through such treatment provides a physiological "massage" that helps open clogged vessels.

Where contrast bathing is used in the treatment of an extremity, e.g., a hand or a foot, the injured part may simply be immersed in hot water (about 110° F) for four to six minutes, and then in cold water (about 50° F) for one to four minutes. The treatment should be begun and ended with immersion in hot water.

Light Exercising

Although active exercise should be delayed until it can be performed without pain, it should be started, lightly, as soon as possible after the hot applications have been initiated in order to make sure that none of the injured fibers become "glued" to the healthy fibers to cause permanent adhesions.

Athletes who rest too long while recovering from muscle injuries may lose balance, skill, and muscle tone, or they may wind up with a stiff muscle that might hamper their playing ability. On the other hand, the premature introduction of overly vigorous exercise and massage, before the injured fibers have healed adequately, may induce a recurrence of bleeding and thus delay recovery.

In using exercise following an injury, the athlete should be guided by common sense and his sense of well-being. He should begin his exercise early, but lightly, and increase the amount of exercise from day to day as long as no ill effects are observed.

Galvanic or sinusoidal (electrical) current is sometimes used by doctors to contract muscle fibers — to prevent adhesions and to preserve muscle tone — whenever active exercise must be delayed in the treatment of a muscle injury.

Strapping a pulled muscle is seldom of any real value, since it might restrict circulation and interfere with treatment. In a fresh injury, however, a compression (elastic) bandage is sometimes used between cold applications to curtail swelling.

Whenever a ligamentous strain, a joint injury, or a complete separation (avulsion) occurs in a muscle or tendon, a physician should be employed to guide the injured athlete back to an active status. With simple muscle injuries, however, the speed and degree of an athlete's recovery will depend largely upon "home treatment."

Enzyme Injections

Team physicians sometimes inject sprained ankles and other athletic injuries with such enzymes as hyaluronidase in order to facilitate absorption of the extravasated blood and tissue fluid and to prevent the clogging up of tiny capillaries. Oral enzymes, such as buccal amylase, may also be helpful in reducing inflammation and swelling.

Injured athletes sometimes take pain killers in order to continue playing in an important game. But since it's difficult to judge the severity of an injury until the cumulative effects of the swelling are observed for several hours, it's usually best to take the injured boy out of the game and apply a cold pack until the injury can be examined by a doctor.

All swollen joints should be brought to the attention of a physician, whether there's been any obvious injury or not. Failure to aspirate a badly swollen knee or ankle could result in the formation of fibrin, which could permanently stiffen the joint.

An improperly treated muscle injury may not only sideline an athlete for a full season, but may also cause a bone formation in the thick, unabsorbed, fibrous tissue formations which may require surgery later on. That's why it's essential to make full use of the basic methods of treatment and then seek the advice of an expert.

Long-range treatment of various types of injuries (in different muscles) will vary from case to case; this article merely scratches the surface. The coach should get a good book on athletic injuries and study it in his spare time.

Summary

Whenever a muscle injury occurs, a cold pack should be applied immediately; if the injury appears to be serious, the cold treatment should be continued off and on for 24 to 36 hours.

After 36 to 48 hours, heat may be applied if it doesn't cause pain, throbbing, or further black and blue discoloration.

Although cold should be used to curtail bleeding and swelling in fresh injuries, it shouldn't be used longer than 48 hours, since it retards healing by restricting the circulation.

Light massage and muscle contraction can usually be started with the application of heat. If no pain or ill-effects are observed, active exercise may be made progressively more vigorous until the muscle is back to normal.

"Charley Horse"

Charles N. Darden

The term "Charley horse" is a common colloquialism referring to certain muscular injuries. While authorities differ on the exact nature of a "Charley horse," most of them agree it's a contusion or bruise resulting from a blow — the most frequent site of injury being the quadriceps femoris on the anterior thigh.

Since (a) there's so much confusion about "Charley horse," (b) it's such a common injury, and (c) it can be painful and debilitating, it follows that a comprehensive treatise on it, covering anatomy, etiology, pathology, prognosis, treatment, complications, and preventative measures, can prove extremely valu· able to coaches and trainers.

Anatomy of Thigh

As a starting point, it's essential to obtain a clear mental picture and understanding of the anatomy and functions of the thigh. A review of a standard text on anatomy is indicated, with particular stress on the femur and its related joints, the quadriceps, and the sartorious muscle.

The femur is the longest and strongest bone in the body. Proximally, it joins the pelvis to form the hip joint. Distally, it joins the tibia to form the knee joint. Thorndike points out that while almost 12% of all athletic injuries occur in the thigh and femoral fractures are quite possible, breaks of the femur are exceedingly rare. He indicates this may be partially due to the protection offered by large tense muscles over the bone.

The sartorius is the longest muscle in the body, being narrow and ribbonlike. It arises from the anterior superior iliac spine and the notch just below it, passes downward obliquely across the upper and anterior part of the thigh, and inserts on the medial aspect of the tibia. Its action is chiefly flexion of the hip.

The quadriceps femoris includes the four remaining muscles on the front of the thigh. The rectus femoris has its origin from the ilium and runs superficially down the middle of the thigh. The other three lie in immediate contact with the body of the femur, which they cover from the trachanters to the condyles.

The lateral portion is called the vastus lateralis; the portion of the medial side of the femur is called the vastus medialis; and the portion of the front of the femur located beneath the rectus femoris is called the vastus intermedius. Vastus lateralis and vastus medialis have small origins from the femur just below the hip joint, but it's important to note the extensive origin of vastus intermedius. The

Reprinted with permission from *Scholastic Coach,* January 1962.

deep vastus intermedius arises from the front and lateral surfaces of the upper two-thirds of the femur.

The tendons of the four different portions of the quadriceps unite at the lower part of the thigh, so as to form a single tendon which inserts into the base of the patella and indirectly into the tuberiosity of the tibia. The chief action of the quadriceps femoris is strong extension of the knee. The rectus femoris also helps flex the thigh.

Within the thigh are also located the usual fascial sheaths, nerves, blood vessels, and lymphatic vessels. A group of lymph nodes are located in the inguinal region.

Etiology

A "Charley horse" results from an external blow on the front of the thigh, producing a contusion. Despite protective padding, "Charley horses" occur rather frequently in football and less frequently in basketball, soccer, lacrosse, and other sports. The traumatic blow is usually the result of a strong shoulder block by an opponent, although a knee or foot may occasionally be the cause. In basketball or soccer, the opponent's knee would most likely be the causative factor.

Stevens and Phelps state that the injury occurs while the muscles are in contraction. Bilik, however, contends that the trauma occurs when the muscles are relaxed.

Pathology

A hard blow on the thigh produces a contusion, or bruise, with extensive damage to all underlying muscles, tendons, blood vessels, lymphatic vessels, and nerves. In severe cases, the periosteum, or outer layers of the bone, may be damaged. Blood vessels and capillaries are ruptured, resulting in hemorrhage into the tissues. Considerable exudation of liquids also occurs in response to the tissue damage.

The pressure of these exudates on the sensory nerve endings produces pain; and motor nerves respond to this stimulation by contraction of the muscle fibers, resulting in muscle spasm. A hematoma is often formed. A hematoma is "a focalized extravasation of blood, which soon clots to form a solid mass and readily becomes encapsulated by connective tissue." It may be of such size as to form a visible or palpable tumorlike swelling.

Pain and loss of function of the part are evident, and continued activity may cause additional damage and hemorrhage, with resultant increase in the length of the recovery period.

Thorndike points out the four stages of repair which usually take place. They are hemorrhage, hematoma formation, hematoma absorption, and repair of tissue.

Initial treatment is chiefly aimed at controlling the amount of hemorrhage and subsequent hematoma formation. Subsequent treatment is mainly aimed at the absorption of the hematoma and extravasations, and the repair of the damaged tissues.

Prognosis

Prognosis depends on the severity of damage to the tissues and the size of the hematoma mass, along with the promptness and perseverance of treatment.

With a non-severe type of contusion, the athlete will usually carry on with only a slight awareness of discomfort. It's not until after the game that he notices a stiffening at the site of injury and a difficulty of motion. The athlete with the non-severe "Charley horse" will usually miss little, if any, playing time, but the injured site should be treated and protected for some time in order to prevent another injury to this area. "A second blow may do a great deal of harm and may even cause permanent disability."

With a moderately severe "Charley horse," the player can usually return to action in one to two weeks if efficient treatment is carried out immediately. With correct treatment, the prognosis for complete recovery is good.

Severe "Charleys" may be disabling for a longer period of time. "The severity varies, and with it the degree of disability."

Treatment

Acute Stage.

The chief aim in the immediate treatment of a "Charley horse" is to prevent as much hemorrhage and hematoma formation as possible. There are several accepted methods to accomplish this. The immediate treatment should consist of rest, compression, ice, and elevation of the extremity.

After the injury, bleeding within the muscle will continue until the pressure inside the injured region is equal to the blood pressure. To reduce the amount of swelling that will occur, it's important to apply immediate compression to the muscle so as to reduce bleeding as much as possible, and to facilitate venous and lymphatic drainage. A piece of sponge rubber should be placed over the injured site, and the thigh wrapped snugly with a four-inch elastic bandage.

After the compression bandage has been fixed, the injured athlete should be placed in a supine position with the leg slightly elevated. This slight elevation will tend to decrease arterial flow and increase venous and lymphatic flow. Cold applications should be applied to the injured site and adjacent areas for at least

30 minutes. A short cold application exerts a vasoconstricting and pain relieving effect in the immediate treatment of contusions and hematomas.

An effective method of cold application is chipped ice wrapped in towels. Ice bags are another method of application. The cold application shouldn't be so cold as to be uncomfortable. In severe contusions, the cold should be continued for several hours after the accident.

After the injured athlete has been treated with cold applications, the wet elastic bandage and sponge should be replaced with a dry bandage and sponge. He should then be instructed to rest the injured thigh as much as possible until the following day, keeping the leg in the horizontal or slightly elevated position. This is to prevent further hemorrhage and give the ruptured blood vessels time to heal through natural body processes.

If the injury is of a mild nature, the athlete should then be transported to his quarters. If the injury is of a moderate or severe nature, he should be taken to the team physician's office. The coach or trainer may administer immediate first aid, but it's of the utmost importance that subsequent treatment be under the guidance of a physician.

Stone stresses the use of ice and compression for longer period of time — from 24 hours to four days after the injury. "We do not feel that it is sufficient to apply ice for a half hour or an hour.... In rather severe injuries, we find that it is necessary to keep the patient at rest and in ice packs and compressions for as long as three or four days."

Bilik adheres to a more spartan treatment. His prescription would be, "I want you to walk around this field for one solid hour, at a moderate pace, but keep going even though there be discomfort." He emphasizes that "walking through" the injury will prevent the organizations of an organized hematoma and hasten and make more thorough the healing of soft tissue injuries. He indicates this is particularly true of the mild and moderate forms of bruises.

Cramer, Boughton, and Cramer believe the immediate treatment should be to stretch the injured area while the athlete is still warm. They feel this stretch will prevent muscular contraction, as well as help retard internal hemorrhage because it increases surface pressure over the injury. They would take the athlete to the training room, remove his clothing, stretch the area, and then apply the ice pack for 30-45 minutes.

No heat or massage should be used in this acute stage of the injury, as this will tend to aggravate the injury and increase the circulation and subsequent swelling and hematoma formation.

Convalescent Stage

Again it should be emphasized that all subsequent treatment should be under the guidance of a physician.

With proper treatment, hemorrhage at the injured site should have ceased within the 24 hour period after the injury. Treatment should then be directed at hastening the absorption of the hematoma and the repair of damaged tissues by increasing the circulation and preventing further injury to the injured site. This end is accomplished by the use of heat, massage, graduated active exercises, and certain protective measures.

After the acute stage, some form of heat should be used daily on the thigh. This is employed for the improvement of circulation, the relief of pain, and as an introduction to massage and exercise. The heat should be of moderate intensity and comfortable at all times — avoiding the common tendency to use heat at too high an intensity — for about 30 minutes duration.

Heating Methods

Preferred methods of heating are hot towels, hydrocallator packs (chemical hot packs which emit moist heat for about 30 minutes), diathermy, or paraffin baths (a paraffin and oil mixture which can be "painted" on in layers over the thigh). The whirlpool bath at 105°-110° Fahrenheit offers a combination of heating and hydro-massage.

In the hands of an experienced and qualified operator, ultrasonic radiation may induce deep heat as well as provide a "cavitational" effect, tending to disintegrate and disperse the hematoma formation. Some feel that research in the medical usage of ultrasonics has been incomplete and would refrain from its usage at the present time.

Massage may be begun after the acute stage, usually after 24 hours. It should be preceded by heat, and some type of lubricant such as mineral oil or olive oil should be used. The entire leg should be massaged, using stroking-type of movement (effleurage).

But massage of the thigh should be light and in the area of the contusion, never on the actual contusion. Meanwell and Rockne point out that massage over the injured site, especially in the early stages of convalescence, will interfere with the processes of repair and may again cause bleeding. Thorndike also warns of the danger of massage over the contusion itself. In potential cases of myositis ossificans traumatica (or, simply stated, ossifying hematoma), rubbing irritates and stimulates the production of greater calcification.

The strokes should be from a little above the injured site toward the inguinal lymph nodes. This serves to empty venous and lymphatic channels, assuring more rapid absorption from the injured site.

The wearing of the elastic bandage should be continued between treatments. This affords a sort of "self-massage," and also increases the efficiency of the venous system. Cramer, Boughton, and Cramer advocate the use of an analgesic pack, which is composed of a thin layer of analgesic balm over the injury, covered by a layer of cotton, and wrapped snugly with an elastic bandage. This furnishes a low-grade heat throughout the day, along with the elastic bandage treatment. Andel reports good results with the use of this pack.

As soon as coaptation and adherence begin in the injury, active motion should be started. A graduated program of active exercises may be started a day or two following the trauma, except in the most severe cases. Active motion as soon as possible is indicated to resolve the edema and extravasation, and to prevent the formation of adhesions and fibrosis.

Lymph exuded after the injury and during the process of inflammation will have a tendency to coagulate and adhere to the adjoining surfaces of muscles, tendons, and fascia. In the latter stages of repair, new tissue will tend to become fibrous and to contract, forming bands which bind adjacent surfaces together, with resultant limitation of motion.

Exercise should proceed gradually within the limits of discomfort, and should progress from active flexion and extension of the knee following heat and massage treatments, to walking, to jogging, to running at full speed, and finally to return to competition with adequate padding over the injury to prevent re-injury.

When the injured athlete regains complete function of the leg, he may be allowed to return to competition, but a protective covering should be used for at least 10 days. A repetition of the injury might have a much more serious pathological sequence. The protective pad should be composed of foam rubber (one-half inch thick) and a hard thigh pad. The rubber should be placed on the thigh, with an air space cut over the injured site. The thigh pad is placed over the rubber.

The attending physician may wish to use one of the newer pharmaceutical preparations as an aid in the convalescent treatment. Enzyme therapy, either orally or intramuscularly, is purported to be of value in the treatment of contusions and hematomas, serving to hasten resolution of the swelling and ecchymosis.

A controlled study of the Texas A. & M. football team in 1956 and 1957 seems to indicate that the use of a water-soluble citrus bioflavonoids compound in capsule form was of value as a prophylatic measure in decreasing the incidence and severity of bruises, hematomas, strains, and sprains. The four doctors conducting the study felt the results warranted continued use of these capsules in 1958. This therapy was directed at restoring and maintaining the integrity of the capillary wall structure.

An example of a treatment regime for a moderate severe "Charley horse" in the convalescent stage might be as follows: Begin by using hydrocallator packs, massage, and graduated active exercises twice daily (morning and afternoon). Use an elastic bandage after the morning treatment, and an analgesic pack after the afternoon session. After a few days, ultra-sound may be substituted for the hydrocallator packs in the afternoon treatment.

If the "Charley horse" shows no improvement or worsens after several days of treatment, the athlete should be returned to the attending physician. Myositis ossificans traumatica must be suspected as the "insidious villain." This condition is discussed in the following section.

Complications

Myositis ossificans traumatica (ossifying hematoma) may be an interesting sequela of a deep muscle contusion. It occurs most often in the vastus intermedius, because of its vast origin from the femur. In the original trauma, tendinous insertions may be pulled from the bone, whereby a few bone cells are loosened to float in the hematoma.

During the convalescent stage, these bone cells proliferate and lay down calcification in the hematoma formation. Generally, X-rays won't reveal this ossification process until three weeks following the trauma. A deep muscle contusion which doesn't respond to the usual treatment after four or five days should be suspected of being a potential myositis ossificans traumatica.

The patient with a suspected ossifying hematoma should be immediately referred back to the attending physician. The usual treatment is rest and heat, with elevation of the involved part. No massage or friction should be allowed around the site of the injury, as this tends to aggravate the injury and promote calcification. Later, gradual active exercise may be started. Some calcified hematomas are absorbed with perfect functional results, while others become chronic and leave a residual disability. Surgery is occasionally indicated.

Dr. Thorndike treated 18 cases of myositis ossificans traumatica at Harvard College over a nine-year period.

A second blow on an original hematoma could possibly lead to the detachment of an embolus, a potentially dangerous situation. An embolus is a clot which moves through the blood vessels. The peril lies in that the embolus may become lodged in certain places within the body which may prove dangerous, such as the heart.

Stevens and Phelps mention that occasionally thrombophlebitis may result from a single serious contusion, but that it's usually the result of repeated injuries over a period of time. In this condition, the veins become blocked with a blood clot, resulting in inflammation or pain and swelling of the leg.

Preventative Measures

The adage, "An ounce of prevention is worth a pound of cure," is applicable to "Charley horses." The coach, trainer, team physician, and athlete should be constantly on the alert for possible preventative measures.

In football, the quality and proper fit of the thigh pad are important.

Stevens and Phelps point out that players cannot be depended on to properly fit or place their own pads, and must be constantly checked by the coach or trainer. The most common fault in fitting seems to be not wearing the pads high enough. The pads should cover as much of the anterior and lateral thighs as possible, and still allow the player to assume the proper stances. The pads should have an inner layer of resilient rubber to help absorb the shock.

Benches, chairs, and other equipment and apparatus shouldn't be left where a boy might run into them.

Summary

"Charley horse" is a colloquial expression that usually signifies a bruise or contusion to the front of the thigh. Often a hematoma is formed.

In its acute phase (usually with the first 24-hour period after the injury, except in the most severe cases), treatment is directed chiefly at prevention of hemorrhage and hematoma formation. Preferred methods of accomplishing this are compression, ice, rest, and elevation of the involved area. No heat or massage should be used at this time. Cramer, Boughton, and Cramer suggest a technique of immediately putting the anterior thigh muscles on a stretch. Bilik believes in "walking through" the injury.

A coach or trainer may apply first aid, but subsequent treatment should be under the guidance of a physician, except for the very mild bruises.

In the convalescent phase, treatment should consist of heat, massage around the contusion (not directly over the injured site), graduated active exercise, elastic bandage application, and protection against re-injury. Ultra sound and analgesic packs are other suggested methods of treatment. The attending physician may wish to use other therapeutic means.

The object of treatment is to increase circulation, promote absorption, accelerate the processes of repair, prevent adhesions and fibrosis, relieve pain and muscle spasm, restore function, and prevent re-injury. The athlete shouldn't be allowed to return to competition until he's regained complete function of the leg, then a protective padding should be worn over the site of injury some time.

Myositis ossificans traumatica is a rather frequent complication of "Charley horses." Less frequent complications are thrombophlebitis and emboli.

Stress should be placed on the prevention of "Charley horses" in football by the proper fitting and placement of adequate thigh pads. Benches and other obstacles into which the athlete may collide should be removed from the playing area.

One difficulty that always arises in the preparation of a paper of this type is determining the level of knowledge of the potential readers. Since this paper was prepared specifically for coaches, physical educators, and trainers, an attempt was made to present the material at this level of comprehension.

REFERENCES

Books

1. Bilik, S.E. *The Trainers' Bible.* New York: T.J. Reed and Co., 1948.
2. *Blakiston's New Gould Dictionary.* New York: The Blakiston Co., 1949.
3. Cramer, Frank, L.L. Boughton, and Charles Cramer. *A Training Room Manual.* Gardner, Kan.: Cramer Athletic Products, 1945.
4. Featherstone, Donald F. *Sports Injuries Manual for Trainers and Coaches.* London: Nicholas Kay, 1954.
5. Goss, Charles May, ed. *Gray's Anatomy of the Human Body*, 26th Ed. Philadelphia: Lea and Febiger, 1954.
6. Grant, J.C. Boileau. *An Atlas of Anatomy*, 4th Ed. Baltimore: The Williams and Wilkins Co., 1956.
7. Kovacs, Richard. *Electrotherapy and Light Therapy*, 6th Ed. Philadelphia: Lea and Febiger, 1949.
8. Lloyd, Frank S., George G. Deaver, and Floyd R. Eastwood. *Safety in Athletics – The Prevention and Treatment of Athletic Injuries.* Philadelphia: W.B. Saunders Co., 1939.
9. Meanwell, Walter E., and Knute K. Rockne. *Training Conditioning and the Care of Injuries.* Madison, Wis.: No publisher listed, 1931.
10. Stevens, Marvin Allen, and Winthrop Morgan Phelps. *The Control of Football Injuries.* New York: A.S. Barnes and Co., 1933.
11. Thorndike, Augustus. *Athletic Injuries, Prevention, Diagnosis and Treatment*, 2nd Ed. Philadelphia: Lea and Febiger, 1942.
12. Wells, Katherine F., *Kinesiology*, 2nd Ed. Philadelphia: W.B. Saunders Co., 1955.

Articles

13. Andel, Buck. "Charley Horse." Pamphlet by the *National Athletic Trainers Association.*
14. Atsatt, R.F. "The High School Football Team Physician." *California Medicine* 87 (October 1957): 264-265.
15. Harrison, R.H., and R.H. Harrison, III, and others. "Athletic Contact Injuries." *Clinical Medicine* 5 (June 1958): 787-790.
16. O'Donaghue, Don H. "General Principles in Treatment of Injuries to Athletes." *Journal of American Medical Association* 171 (21 November 1959): 132-135.
17. Rawlinson, Kenneth B. "Athletic Training, Protective Equipment, and Protective Support." *Journal of American Medical Association* 171 (21 November 1959): 146-148.
18. Slocum, David B. "The Mechanics of Common Football Injuries." *Journal of American Medical Association* 170 (August 1959): 1640-1646.
19. Stone, Frank P. "Athletic Injuries." *The Nebraska State Medical Journal* 42 (September 1957): 430-435.
20. Thorndike, Augustus. "Myositis Ossificans Traumatica." *The Journal of Bone and Joint Surgery* 22 (April 1940): 315-323.
21. Wedlick, Leigh T. "Sports Injuries." *The Medical Journal of Australia* 46 (13 June 1959): 801-802.

Blisters—No Problem

A. G. Edwards

In late June of 1924 Calvin Coolidge, Jr., finished a spirited game of tennis and noticed he had a rather painful blister on his big toe. Two weeks later on July 7 the President's son died of blood poisoning brought on by this relatively insignificant injury.

While the problem of blisters in athletics today rarely, if ever, reaches such tragic proportions; nevertheless, it is a concern to all trainers and athletes. Improper treatment of a blister can remove an athlete from competition for a critical period of time.

At the present time it is unnecessary for an athlete to be incapacitated for any period of time due to a blister. Conscientious trainers and coaches can use simple and inexpensive methods to forestall any complication when blisters strike their athletes. Mr. Jim Hunt, trainer at the University of Michigan, developed a method of treatment which is now in wide use.

Perhaps the first step in any program should be an accent on the prevention of blisters. This need not be time-consuming and with some simple instructions each athlete can take care of his own feet. A preventive method to use is as follows:

1. Put a good coat of tincture of benzoin on the problem areas. Usually this is placed on the ball of the foot, the back of the heel, and the big toe. Be sure to cover a large area. We do not believe this method has anything to do with getting the skin tough; it is a preparation for step three.

2. Allow the tincture of benzoin to dry.

3. Apply inch and a half tape to the susceptible areas.

4. Because of the contour of the foot, there will be a gap in the tape. . . . There will also be one in the tape on the toe. These gaps should be pinched together and cut off so they will not wrinkle and cause additional blisters and skin irritation.

The simple theory behind this method is to transfer the friction of the shoe to the tape and not the skin. The most important step is applying a good coat of benzoin. Many athletes entering the Ferris State College program say they have never been through a season without blisters. They relate that often a number of practice days, and, most important, competitive opportunities, have been missed due to blisters. This is especially true of track athletes because so many do not wear socks.

Athletes at Ferris who use the preceding treatment report no blister problems. It does not cut down the number of blisters; it cuts them out completely.

Reprinted with permission from *Athletic Journal*, June 1968.

Occasionally, of course, blisters do occur — a new boy comes out late or the careless athlete does not use proper prevention. Again, this should present no difficulty for the informed trainer or coach and these athletes should not miss even a single day of practice. The procedure to use in the treatment is as follows:

1. Cleanse the area with soap and hot water and then cover the entire area with a 3 percent solution of hydrogen peroxide.

2. If the blister has broken open, remove the dead skin with sterile tweezers and scissors. If the blister is closed, it must be opened and the fluid removed. A trainer should obtain permission from the team physician to open the blister and remove the fluid or let the physician do it.

3. After the blister has been opened and the fluid drained, all dead skin should be removed.

4. Use a cotton-topped application, and swab the area with hydrogen peroxide.

5. Apply an antiseptic to the blistered area. Many good antiseptics can be used which have a minimal astringent effect. This, of course, is necessary because the area is very tender.

6. Cover the area surrounding the blister with tincture of benzoin.

7. Apply inch and a half tape directly over the blister. A tape that is porous and has a zinc oxide backing will give better results.

8. Pinch together the gaps and cut.

After completing this treatment, it is important that the athlete receive careful instruction. The tape should remain on the treated area from three to four days depending on the severity of the blister. It should not be removed for any reason.

Once this *friction shield* has been placed between the most tender area and the shoe, the athlete can practice that very day. Athletes at Ferris who have been treated with this procedure performed competitively on the same day.

When the three- to four-day period has elapsed, the tape should be removed gently and a new layer of skin will have grown over the blistered area. It is no longer necessary to leave the tape on continually, but the healing area should be protected during the workouts.

Hunt's simple yet complete method of treating blister problems is unequaled for effectiveness. The amount of time lost through aggravating injuries to competing athletes will be, at the very least, minimal and probably non-existent.

While modern drugs have certainly brought protection to the serious complications that blisters can produce, such as blood poisoning which struck down Coolidge's son, no secondary treatment should be necessary if trainers follow the precautions and treatment described.

Soft Tissue Injuries

Richard E. Carr

Technically speaking, any injury that does not involve bone is a soft tissue injury; however, we will concern ourselves with the soft tissue injuries which are commonly known as wounds. Various forms of wounds are common in athletics and must be treated effectively in order to prevent infection and to hasten as much as possible the healing process which takes place. Wounds are classified as abrasions, lacerations, incisions, and punctures.

Abrasions

Abrasions are also known as slide burns, grass burns, and strawberries. They are usually not deep, but may cover large surfaces of the skin. These wounds usually do not bleed much, but later on will ooze and cause the dressing to stick.

These abrasions should be cleaned thoroughly and a dressing applied with a non-stick material if it is available. We use Nitrotan followed by strawberry ointment and covered by a telfa pad which is non-stick. Soap and water, tincture of green soap or Phisohex, a surgical soap, can be used to cleanse these wounds.

Lacerations

Lacerations are a tearing of the flesh and are not common in athletics although they do occur. First aid treatment consists of the control of hemorrhage, cleansing, and the application of a sterile dressing.

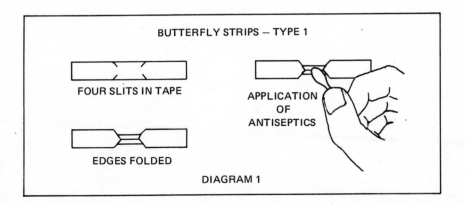

BUTTERFLY STRIPS — TYPE 1

FOUR SLITS IN TAPE

APPLICATION OF ANTISEPTICS

EDGES FOLDED

DIAGRAM 1

Reprinted with permission from *Athletic Journal,* January 1969.

Incisions

An incision is an even wound such as a surgeon makes in the flesh when performing surgery. About the same number of these occur as do the laceration type of wound and first aid is the same.

The control of hemorrhage or bleeding is facilitated by the use of a pressure bandage and the application of cold.

Diagrams 1 and 2 show the butterfly tape that is useful in closing lacerations or incisions which are not severe enough to require sutures. Diagram 1 shows how to make the butterfly strips and Diagram 2 the ready-prepared sterile bandages in the three different sizes.

Puncture

Next to abrasions, puncture wounds are the most common in athletics and by far the most dangerous.

These puncture wounds occur from football cleats, baseball spikes, and track spikes. They are usually small on the surface, but penetrate deep into the tissue. Puncture wounds do not bleed freely and are hard to cleanse thoroughly.

First aid is the same as it is for lacerations and incisions, but the most important thing is that these wounds be seen by a physician and a tetanus shot given if the player has not had one within one year.

Contusions or bruises are not wounds, but are soft tissue injuries and should not be neglected. The application of ice and pressure is the early treatment followed by heat and protective padding.

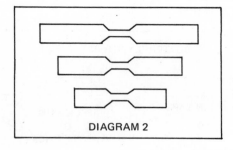

DIAGRAM 2

Heat Stress in Physical Activity

Dr. Avery Harvill

As physical educators and coaches, we pride ourselves on the accomplishments achieved in the teaching of skills, the development of fine athletes, and winning teams. In accomplishing these desired objectives, we have had to recognize and utilize specific physiological principles and have worked diligently to incorporate them into our practice schedules. We have, however, in our rush for success overlooked or ignored some very important principles that have, on occasion, erupted with tragic consequences.

Every year far too many would-be athletes, following the dictates of the teacher or coach, are carried from the field to the hospital emergency room, a step away from death, due to loss of vital body fluids or a temperature of 108°. The tragedy of these situations is that they should not occur at all. By simply following a few simple safety procedures, the physical education classes and athletic teams can participate safely and more effectively during hot weather than at present.

Let us look first at the process utilized by the body to regulate its temperature.

The body's temperature is relatively consistent with little day to day variation. Body heat is generated primarily by muscle activity and to a lesser extent by metabolic action. The methods for reducing body temperature are quite effective when the environmental temperature is below skin temperature. Twenty percent of the body heat is lost by radiation, conduction, and convection, and nearly 30 percent by evaporation from respiratory tract and skin (1).

When the environmental temperature rises above skin temperature, the body will actually take on heat through radiation, conduction, and convection rather than losing it, and must depend entirely on evaporation for cooling. As the humidity rises to the point where it approaches 100 percent, the evaporation approaches zero, and the body perspires freely but cools little. The point where moderate exertion results in a steady rise in body temperature is referred to as the death line (2). The individual's ability to perspire and the air's ability to take on more moisture becomes a life-and-death matter.

A growing number of researchers have studied the problem of acclimatizing individuals to heat as we have so often done in altitude acclimatization. It is found that the heat acclimatized person starts to perspire earlier, puts out more perspiration per unit of time, his perspiration contains much less salt, and by changes in circulation, he gets more blood to the surface with less work load on the heart (3).

Reprinted with permission from *Athletic Journal,* June, 1967.

As an individual perspires, he loses water and salt. If this process is allowed to continue for a period of time unaided, dehydration will result as well as a loss of essential body salt. Research indicates that a 6 percent loss of body weight will result in a 15 percent loss by volume of blood plasma (4).

The intake of water is not the only solution since the body is unable to control water loss in the absence of sufficient salt (5). Water relieves dehydration but lowers the concentration of salt in the extra-cellular fluid, resulting in heat cramps.

Since salt is essential for health and the avoidance of the adverse effects of heat, most coaches and teachers must administer extra salt in specified quantities. One writer (6) recommends the administration of from 6 to 12 five-grain salt tablets per day depending on the weight of the player, Karpovich (7) and de Vries (8) indicate that under the most severe conditions of the tropics, an intake of 13 to 17 grams of salt a day is sufficient. This is equivalent to 3¼ to 4¼ teaspoons of salt or 20 to 26 five-grain salt tablets.

All players should be weighed before and after practice each day. Any player losing more than 3 percent of his body weight during a practice session should have his salt and water intake increased (9). Herbert de Vries (10) feels that the loss of 2 or 3 pounds is sufficient to call for an increase in liquid and salt.

The question now arises as to the process of heat acclimating an individual and in deciding on the procedure allowed for fluid intake.

Let us look first at the acclimation process. Four authors indicated that the time required for heat acclimation should be five days (11), two workouts a day for ten days (12), five to eight days (13), and a minimum of four weeks (14). While there is a wide variation in the length of time necessary for heat acclimation, all authors are in agreement that such a period is necessary. It seems logical to conclude that the acclimation period should be a minimum of five days, with ten days tending to be desirable.

The acclimation process should generally adhere to the following procedure: Work easily for moderate periods, approximately 30 minutes, with adequate periods of rest between, normally 20 minutes. During these rest periods water and salt should be administered. Workouts should be performed initially in shorts and T-shirts with the addition of protective equipment, light contact and a jersey added after a minimum of five days. All equipment should be as light in weight as possible, light in color, and permit free circulation of air (shirt-tail out, short sleeves, loose fitting collar).

During the acclimation period, in particular, the participants should be watched for signs of heat stress such as headache, excessive redness, cessation of perspiration, dizziness, and being sick at the stomach. The coach should be aware of these symptoms during any practice session but especially so during periods of hot, humid weather.

While research indicates that the intake of large quantities of water does not adversely affect an individual's performance (15, 16), most coaches are hesitant about giving their charges free access to the water bucket.

It is generally thought that during practice a rest break should be taken every 30 minutes and 10 ounces of salt water consumed. During the first week the salt concentration should be 4 or 5 teaspoons per gallon, reduced to 3 teaspoons for the next week, and then 2 teaspoons until cool weather (17).

Between practice sessions athletes should seek to cool off and take on extra salt and liquids. Diet is also of some concern. Foods that are high in water content are recommended while protein in the diet should be decreased due to heat formation created by protein digestion (18).

The hazardous connection between temperature and humidity has been mentioned previously. The question arises as to how a coach or teacher can decide the type of practice or class activities that can safely be held. A sophomore football player in one of our large cities died after participating in a scrimmage when the temperature on the field was 114 degrees, even though practice was held late in the day.

The necessary information concerning temperature and humidity can and should be gathered on the field at 30-minute intervals during a practice since conditions change rapidly and vary from place to place. This measurement can be taken from a psychrometer, an instrument with a wet and a dry thermometer.

The readings on the psychrometer may be interpreted as follows:

1. When the temperature is below 80° and relative humidity less than 70 percent, no special precautions are required.

2. When the temperature is between 80° and 90° with a relative humidity of less than 70 percent, the coach or teacher must observe his players carefully for signs of heat stress.

3. When the temperature is between 80° and 90° with a relative humidity higher than 70 percent or with a temperature of 90° or 100° and humidity under 70 percent, frequent rest periods must be observed, wet shirts changed, and other clothing and pads kept at a minimum.

4. At temperatures between 90° and 100° with a relative humidity over 70 percent, or when the temperature is above 100° and there is any humidity, practice should be postponed or conducted for a limited time in extremely light clothing and with abundant rest periods (19).

REFERENCES

1. Karpovich, P.V. *Physiology of Muscular Activity*, p. 209.
2. Buttram, W.R., Jr. *Prevention of Heat Illness*, Chattanooga, Hamilton County Medical Society, August 1966, unpublished paper.
3. Buttram, op. cit.
4. Adolph, E.F., and others. *Physiology of Man in the Desert*.

5. Morehouse, F., *Physiology of Exercise.*
6. Ryan, A.J. "The Response of Athletes to Heat Stress." *Annual Safety Education Review*, 1966, p. 17.
7. Karpovich, op. cit.
8. de Vries, H.A. *Physiology of Exercise*, p. 275.
9. Ryan, op. cit., p. 17.
10. de Vries, op. cit., p. 276.
11. Ibid., p. 277.
12. Buttram, op. cit.
13. Karpovich, op. cit., p. 216.
14. Ryan, op. cit., p. 16.
15. Little, C.C., Strayhorn, H., and Miller, A.T. "Effects of Water Ingestion on Capacity for Exercise." *Research Quarterly*, December 1949, pp. 398-401.
16. Mathews, D.C. "More on Heat Stroke." *Medicine and Sports Newsletter.* Rystan, Mount Vernon, New York, October 1964.
17. Buttram, op. cit.
18. de Vries, op. cit., p. 277.
19. Ryan, op. cit., pp. 16-17.

Suggested Levels of First Aid Instruction

CONTENT	LEVELS
Breathing Maintenance and Restoration Bleeding Control How to Summon Assistance Care for the Casualty	**I** LIFE-SAVING TECHNIQUES (For everyone, starting with school children)
Work of the Human Body General Directions of First Aid Respiratory and Cardiac Resuscitation Bleeding Control and Care of Wounds Shock Control and Casualty Management Unconsciousness and Sudden Illness Poisons, Drugs, Bites, Stings, Plants Fractures and other Skeletal Injuries	**II** BASIC FIRST AID (For those desiring to have a basic first aid knowledge for protection of self and family and voluntary service.)
Review of the above with Greater Detail Advanced Bandaging and Splinting Rescue and Transportation Special Wounds and Emergencies Psychiatric Emergencies Maternity Emergencies Survival and Disaster Procedures First Aid Kits and Supplies	**III** ADVANCED FIRST AID (For those needing or desiring comprehensive first aid training.) Includes the above in greater detail plus the content to the left.
Use of Oxygen and Resuscitators Use of Splints, Stretchers, and Lifting Gear Use of Cutting and Rescue Equipment Ambulance Equipment and Supplies First Aid Station Supplies General Rescue and Retrieval Techniques Mountain Rescue Techniques Sea and Water Rescue Techniques Special Emergencies for Young and Old Sports Injuries Industrial Accidents Disaster and Mass Casualty Management Relief Services and Casualty Centers Assistance in Hospital or Casualty Center Accident Investigating and Reporting First Aid Instruction	**IV** SPECIAL FIRST AID REQUIREMENTS (For those who have need of special first aid skills in line with their profession or special activities. At this level the person should be thoroughly familiar with the above and be able to perform the additional skills at the left as required in their work or duties, i.e., expedition or recreation leaders, industrial first-aiders, military corpsmen, police, firemen, ambulance personnel, nurses, and paramedical personnel.)
Tracheostomy and Intubation Oxygen Administration Plasma Transfusions Emergency Amputation Administration of Anesthetics Administration of Emergency Drugs Casualty Management and Follow-Up Organize Group Emergency Medical Services	**V** MEDICAL DOCTORS (Medical Training does not automatically produce a good first-aider. On this level a doctor should be familiar with the above, be able to conduct on-site emergency treatment, and be able to organize emergency medical and health services.)

First Aid Survey

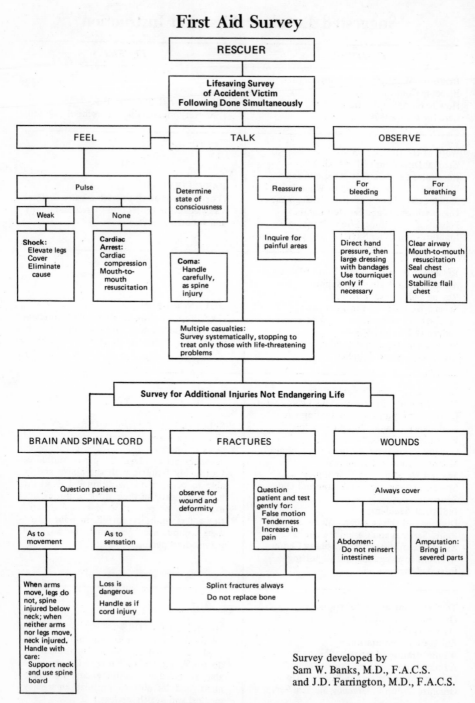

RESCUER

Lifesaving Survey of Accident Victim Following Done Simultaneously

FEEL — **TALK** — **OBSERVE**

Pulse

Weak

None

Shock: Elevate legs Cover Eliminate cause

Cardiac Arrest: Cardiac compression Mouth-to-mouth resuscitation

Determine state of consciousness

Coma: Handle carefully, as spine injury

Reassure

Inquire for painful areas

For bleeding

Direct hand pressure, then large dressing with bandages Use tourniquet only if necessary

For breathing

Clear airway Mouth-to-mouth resuscitation Seal chest wound Stabilize flail chest

Multiple casualties: Survey systematically, stopping to treat only those with life-threatening problems

Survey for Additional Injuries Not Endangering Life

BRAIN AND SPINAL CORD — **FRACTURES** — **WOUNDS**

Question patient

As to movement

As to sensation

When arms move, legs do not, spine injured below neck; when neither arms nor legs move, neck injured. Handle with care: Support neck and use spine board

Loss is dangerous Handle as if cord injury

observe for wound and deformity

Question patient and test gently for: False motion Tenderness Increase in pain

Splint fractures always Do not replace bone

Always cover

Abdomen: Do not reinsert intestines

Amputation: Bring in severed parts

Survey developed by
Sam W. Banks, M.D., F.A.C.S.
and J.D. Farrington, M.D., F.A.C.S.

Reprinted from "Death in a Ditch," Bulletin, May/June, 1967, with permission from the American College of Surgeons.